UNSELF

Transform Your Life By Letting
Go of Who You're Not

DR. OLA ADENIRANYE

Published by

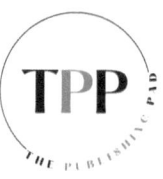

The Publishing Pad
www.thepublishingpad.com

Dedication

Dedicated to you

Praise for *Unself*

"*If you want to break free from the unconscious chains and start living intentionally and with gratitude, this book will help you rewrite your narrative. This is a must-read for anyone who wants to taste the sweet nectar of happiness, being able to return to each passage at any point in their life and find fulfillment.*"
—**Dr. Amanda Moreno,** Psy.D., Clinical Forensic Psychologist

"*As a psychologist, I believe the information and tools offered in this book will help my clients achieve true contentment and be more compassionate of themselves in the process. His user-friendly and no-nonsense approach makes this self-help book one worth delving into. Do yourself a favor and start your journey toward an authentic self.*"
—**Dr. Antoine Saldubehere,** Psy.D., Psychologist In Private Practice, Specializing in Individual and Family Therapy

"*Dr. Ola's UNSELF is a masterclass in personal transformation—clear, insightful, and deeply resonant. There are no stories or fluff here—just clear, focused guidance and thoughtful prompts that help you take inventory of your patterns, assumptions, and internal blocks. Dr. Ola writes with a steady, grounded voice, gently nudging you toward greater self-awareness and freedom. In a world that often rewards performance over presence, UNSELF is a necessary and powerful invitation to come home to yourself.*"
—**Talia Haller,** Future of Health Thought Leader & Speaker

"I completely resonate with Dr. Ola's "HEART" concept. I'm constantly trying to illustrate the importance of this in a sociopolitical environment that overly emphasizes "safe spaces," "boundaries," and "protecting one's peace." These concepts, though well-intentioned, have created an illusion of health and can limit resilience, personal growth, and happiness. Dr. Ola's HEART concept I believe will help individuals break free from this illusion and subsequent fragility, to live more autonomous, competent, and connected lives for achieving and maintaining eudaimonia."

—Dr. Aileen Herlinda Sandoval, Psy.D., Psychologist and Expert Witness on Brain Function and Autism Spectrum Disorder

"*The Unself: Transforming Your Life by Letting Go of Who You're Not!* written by Dr. Olabanji Adeniranye discusses different frameworks that will be helpful for individuals who may have difficulty understanding themselves, and how to transform their identity to their true selves."

—Dr. Tania Hormozi, PsyD, LMFT, Self-published Author, Cooked vs. Uncooked Spaghetti

Table of Contents

"When I look back on my past and think how much time I wasted on nothing, how much time has been lost in futilities, errors, laziness, incapacity to live; how little I appreciated it, how many times I sinned against my heart and soul—then my heart bleeds. Life is a gift, life is happiness, every minute can be an eternity of happiness."

—FYODOR DOSTOEVSKY

Introduction

As a therapist treating patients in different clinical settings for over a decade, I noticed a theme common to all of them: they felt that the world was somewhat alien, foreign, and ambiguous, and that there was no map or how-to guide on how to navigate the depth of its mysteries. This is something I understood and could relate to.

It was my interest in understanding the world, and both my own experience and that of others, that led me to major in psychology. Eventually I became a licensed marriage and family therapist and, later, a psychologist. The world was so confusing to me that I felt like an alien from another planet. I began to wonder: What if I actually were an alien trying to live on Earth? What skills would I need in order to not just survive here, but thrive, flourish, and prosper? I wished I'd been born with those skills, but I had to come to terms with the reality that something was lacking in my approach.

What I could do was pay more attention. I could pay closer attention to what the world was trying to tell me. And if I took heed, I could perhaps change my story—both the past I carried with me and the future I was building.

As I worked with my patients to uncover the source of their suffering and pain, I had an epiphany that struck me like a thunderbolt. This feeling of alienation was a common narrative that took shape into predictable patterns. My patients felt alienated from their thoughts, emotions, and choices; from their family and friends; from their communities. They felt detached and disoriented. The world seemed obtuse and confusing. Some believed they knew what to do but couldn't execute. Some struggled with focus or impulsivity. Others found themselves in classes, jobs, or relationships that brought them no satisfaction. Some of their behaviors, upon deep reflection, seemed absurd to them. "Why did I do that?" they would ask. "Everyone else seems to 'get it,' so why not me? What is wrong with me?"

If you're here, it's likely because a part of you longs for a deeper sense of fulfillment—a life where the dreams in your mind become reality. Perhaps there's an unease you can't quite shake, a wish to relieve that constant, sometimes arbitrary pain, whether physical, mental, or spiritual. You might find yourself caught up in questions that linger but rarely get answered: *Who am I? How did my life turn out this way? Why do these things keep happening to me?* Maybe there are some regrets sprinkled in, too. And let's be honest: who hasn't wished they could turn back time for a second chance at life, but this time armed with a lifetime's worth of insights and perhaps even a bit of omniscience and omnipotence?

A 2023 global survey found that nearly 60% of adults report feeling unfulfilled, often due to a lack of purpose. The external pressures of today's world, such as socioeconomic challenges, geopolitical unrest, and climate concerns, only deepen this sense of disconnection. But external stressors are only part of the picture. Internal struggles related to health, work, family, or relationships layer on top of the world's noise, creating even more tension. It's easy to feel adrift, even for those with a generally positive outlook. When life demands so much of us, chronic stress, anxiety, and self-doubt can take hold, making it difficult to break free from stagnation.

If any of this resonates, you're not alone, and you're not without hope. But the solution you're looking for might not be as straightforward as you'd wish. Instead, what lies ahead is an invitation to undertake a journey: a commitment to deconstruct, examine, and reconstruct yourself. This process is one of gene-deep, continuous self-reflection, a constant journey inward, not to find some elusive and anemic ideal of happiness, but to cultivate a meaningful, dynamic life rooted in clarity and self-awareness. Happiness as it is currently packaged and presented to us is like old-time snake oil, labeled and promoted with false claims and empty promises. What we need is something genuine and enduring.

Becoming a clinician in the mental health field helped me understand that every patient faces challenges centered around the same core issues: their priorities (HEART), the process (TRACE) through which they address these priorities, and their presence (GRACE), the ability to remain balanced and mindful in the face of life's inherent difficulties. It became my life's work to provide people with tools to help them feel less alienated and more connected—authentic, balanced, and at peace.

In a world filled with noise, complexity, and unpredictability, it can feel challenging to separate what's truly important from the clamor that pervades our attention and awareness. Our conditioning, reflected in beliefs, behaviors, and responses, often stems from values and norms that we didn't necessarily choose but have absorbed over time. This kind of conditioning clouds our perception, making us feel like passive passengers on our own journeys. But by peeling back these layers of conditioning, we can reconnect with our authentic selves and uncover a sense of purpose that goes beyond the arbitrary pressures of day-to-day life.

There's an underlying "life script" that governs our actions—beliefs, habits, and choices that, when left unchecked, steer us in predictable directions. Without awareness, we mistake these patterns for fate, but beneath the surface complexity lies a set of simple truths, an underlying structure that influences much of what we experience as chaotic or uncertain.

We're also bombarded with distractions, digital devices, social media, advertising, all competing for our attention. If it feels like your mind is being pulled in every direction, that's because it is. Finding clarity in a world filled with constant, overwhelming noise is both challenging and essential. Unless you have the means to disconnect completely and live off the grid in solitude, finding regular peace can feel impossible.

In the field of leadership studies, the acronym VUCA means volatile, uncertain, complex, and ambiguous. We live in a VUCA world, in which the daily turbulence of the human experience can leave one trapped in an unrelenting cycle of struggle and disillusionment. For some, the tragedy is softened by ignorance, a blissful curse that veils the slow descent into a featureless abyss. For others, awareness is its own torment, as if we are both the architects and spectators of our own unraveling.

There is hope yet. Change is possible. This book outlines a system, a simple yet effective scaffold, to provide the structure you need to see tangible progress. It acknowledges the inevitable challenges, including emotional conflict and cognitive dissonance, but it also equips you with tools to navigate them. These systems are designed to guide you toward finding peace and purpose while helping you envision the next chapter or season of your life.

* * *

This book is your invitation to break free from the unending cycle using frameworks I call HEART, TRACE, and GRACE.

The book is divided into three parts:

- **Part One, "The Foundation,"** will teach you how the HEART system (Health, Enterprise, Authentic Relationships, Recreation and Recovery, and Transcendent Purpose and Meaning) creates coherence by aligning your actions with your core values. You'll also discover how the TRACE process (Time, Resistance, Awareness, Control, and Evolving) supports this alignment, helping you measure meaningful progress where it matters most.
- **Part Two, "The Framework,"** takes a deeper dive into each HEART priority, offering strategies and real-world examples to help you clarify your goals and apply TRACE metrics to achieve them.
- **Part Three, "Putting It All Together,"** will show you how to consolidate your vision, create a cohesive plan for your life, and implement strategies for sustained growth and resilience. We'll also explore the concept of GRACE and the importance of Gratitude, Radical Acceptance, Compassion, and Expectations on the path to living a meaningful, fulfilling life. No matter what challenges arise, you'll be equipped to navigate them with confidence, purpose, and adaptability.

Psychologist Lev Vygotsky introduced the concept of the *zone of proximal development*, where learning builds on what we already know while reaching for the unknown. The HEART, TRACE, and GRACE system in this book is designed to serve as your own zone of proximal development, expanding your current understanding and offering a framework that's both familiar and transformative.

Through the guidance in these pages, I hope you're inspired to take control of your journey, embrace growth, and actively apply the HEART, TRACE, and GRACE frameworks. These tools will empower you to make intentional choices, track meaningful progress, and cultivate lasting transformation.

If you've ever felt disoriented, unsatisfied, or stuck, you're not alone. This book will guide you step by step in cultivating purpose and fulfillment. By making intentional choices that align with your true self, you can create the life you desire. I've witnessed countless individuals shed unworkable parts of their old selves and stories and step into new narratives with a renewed sense of purpose and meaning. It is my hope that these same principles, when applied consistently, will help you transform your own life.

Welcome to *Unself: Transform Your Life by Letting Go of Who You're Not*!

PART ONE:

The Foundation

CHAPTER 1

Redefining Happiness

"In oneself lies the whole world, and if you know how to look and learn, then the door is there and the key is in your hand."[1]

—Jiddu Krishnamurti

If you're reading this book, you are undoubtedly on a quest for more than answers. You're seeking the courage to step into the unknown, to confront the fears that keep you tethered, and to uncover the subtle, quiet patterns shaping your life. This is no ordinary journey. It's a trek where the peaks and valleys of the heart and mind reveal their hidden truths in the shadows they cast. We must go into that darkness, into the fray.

Your yearning for exploration is like that of an astronaut who is driven by a thirst for knowledge as vast as the unknown itself. It's not just about finding meaning; it's about reclaiming the chaos, shaping it into order, and

---

1   Jiddu Krishnamurti, You Are the World: Authentic Report of Talks and Discussions in American Universities, Krishnamurti Foundation India, 1972, p. 148.

uncovering the intricate designs woven into the very fabric of nature, and, by extension, your being.

Yielding to this call into the unknown is a testament to your resilience and your refusal to settle for mediocrity or quiet desperation. It is a call to venture farther, to find not just answers but yourself.

This book will ask something of you. And that is to reflect, to observe, and to watch yourself nonjudgmentally. Imagine yourself as the lens of a hidden device that is recording the patterns of your life when you are at your most oblivious, at your most vulnerable—when you're at the very peak of your creaturely self. What do you see? Would you describe your observations, these patterns, as "happiness"?

Are you happy?

Take a moment to reflect on that question.

Do you know what happiness looks and feels like when it is tailored to fit you? Or is your brand of happiness a prescription with someone else's name on it? After some reflection, whatever your answer is to the question "Are you happy?" will suffice. That's what we're here to address.

Often, we get caught up in what we think of as happiness. Mostly it's an illusion of gossamer built on foundations made of sand. Life can be a frenzy. It is seemingly perpetually chaotic, overwhelming, and overstimulating, leaving us emotionally, mentally, and spiritually undernourished. We're too tired, too busy, too caught up in the speed of the world to realize we're not genuinely happy.

Sometimes, when you do realize the truth of your predicament, the realization arrives uninvited, like an intruder, an overwhelming force that leaves you breathless, as if the very ground beneath you has given way. Other times, it can be a slow burn of discontent that eats away at your existence, leaving your resentment to build until you feel as if your chest might explode. No matter how the realization comes to you, realizing that you're not living an authentic, rich, and meaningful life can be painful.

It's no surprise that when I asked my patients what they sought from therapy, the most common response was simply, "I just want to be happy." These men and women came from all walks of life, all classes and castes. They ranged from people whose lives were ostensibly favored by the gods themselves to the less fortunate who seemed hand-picked to walk through a crucible designed for the biblical character Job himself to traverse.

There was the couple who, after a decade of marriage, had hit a wall after years of sweeping their issues under the rug. There was the serial dater who was unsure whether to pursue a budding romance or return to a former partner with whom they shared a comfortable but complicated history. There was the high-powered professional haunted by impostor syndrome, weighing the stability of a vapid but well-paying job against a longing for something more meaningful. There was the marine, recently retired, with post-traumatic stress disorder who felt lost without the aegis of the uniform. And there was the single parent locked in a bitter custody dispute with a once-beloved partner, struggling to reconcile a past relationship with the demands of the present.

Despite their apparent differences, a familiar theme tied all their responses together: a desire for a joyous life that transcends class, culture, ethnicity, beliefs, or gender. Each one was searching for happiness, the philosopher's stone.

But . . . What Is Happiness?

According to the American Psychological Association (APA), happiness is an emotion of "joy, gladness, satisfaction, and well-being."[2] But happiness goes beyond these terms; it also includes feelings of contentment and *overall* well-being. Some people experience happiness through achievement, while others find it in positive experiences and still others are happy simply in the absence of negative experiences. With happiness defined so differently for each person, it's no wonder the search for it is so complex.

---

2   "Happiness," APA Dictionary of Psychology (website), updated April 19, 2018, https://dictionary.apa.org/happiness/.

A common challenge people face is figuring out exactly what happiness means to them. It's easy to chase fleeting forms of happiness without knowing what will truly satisfy us. Happiness has many forms, and understanding the *quality*, *quantity*, *frequency*, and *duration* of our experiences can have profound effects on our lives.

For instance, consider a lifelong athlete who finds happiness through nutrition and fitness. Their happiness might come from achieving fitness goals, receiving compliments on their appearance, or the sense of purpose they find in daily routines. They may experience long-term happiness through health that sustains them well into old age. This example shows just one way happiness can take on unique and deeply personal forms.

The Quality of Happiness

The quality of happiness we pursue is critical. While a quick burst of pleasure can feel good in the short term, we have to ask: what are the long-term consequences if these pursuits are brief or lack depth?

One of the biggest challenges with all emotions is that they're temporary. Emotions ebb and flow, driven by both external and internal factors. They will remain fleeting unless constantly nurtured or rekindled by something lasting.

When my clients say *I want to be happy*, what they truly mean is that they're searching for fulfillment, wholeness, and freedom from pain. Yet, many people can't easily distinguish this lasting contentment from fleeting pleasure. They're often left chasing a shallow, two-dimensional pseudo-happiness, a cheap fuel that burns too bright and too fast, leaving them wanting more. What they're truly seeking is genuine, authentic contentment, what philosophers call *eudaimonia*.

Eudaimonia: A Deeper Kind of Happiness

Eudaimonia, derived from the Greek *eu-* (good) and *daimon* (spirit), is often defined as "flourishing" or "thriving." It represents a deep sense of well-being, purpose, and contentment that arises from living in alignment with one's true nature and potential. Understanding the concept of eudaimonia requires understanding that there is an experience of lasting fulfillment beyond fleeting happiness.

Eudaimonia goes beyond momentary pleasure and focuses instead on living a virtuous and meaningful life. It springs forth from within and is expressed through a radical, symbiotic engagement with life itself, derived from the synthesis and transcendent understanding of the biopsychosocial experience inherent in being alive.

Eudaimonia is like the ironwood tree deep in the Amazon rainforest, exposed to every element, harsh and otherwise. Its trunk, as hard as an indestructible metal alloy, withstands the test of time, weathering storms and scorching heat. Its root system forges deeper, pushing through the dense soil to access nutrients and stay anchored; its branches reach ever higher to connect with the sun's rays. This tree doesn't just endure the wilderness; it thrives, becoming stronger through each challenge, rooted in resilience and the pursuit of growth.

Pseudo-happiness, on the other hand, is like a delicate houseplant, its vibrant leaves wilting at the slightest change of light, temperature, or moisture. A little too much water, a modest drop in temperature, or even a slight shift in light can send the plant into decline. It survives only in ideal conditions, unable to withstand any disruption. Its growth is shallow, fleeting, and dependent on external factors that often leave it vulnerable when the circumstances shift.

Where eudaimonia deepens in adversity, pseudo-happiness crumbles at the slightest inconvenience. True fulfillment, like the ironwood tree, requires deep roots and the courage to stand tall in the face of life's storms.

Without understanding this, we will continue to misconstrue what authentic eudaimonic happiness means.

Peeling Back the Layers: Hedonic and Eudaimonic Perspectives on Happiness

To understand happiness on a deeper level, let's look at it from two perspectives: *hedonic* and *eudaimonic*.

The word *hedonic* stems from the Greek *hedone*, meaning pleasure. From a hedonic perspective, well-being centers around maximizing pleasure and satisfying desires.[3] *Subjective well-being*, another term for happiness from a hedonic approach, consists of the presence of positive emotional experiences, the absence of negative ones, and a cognitive component, i.e., evaluating one's life as satisfying.[4] In contrast, a eudaimonic perspective of well-being emphasizes living in alignment with one's values and realizing one's fullest potential.[5]

Psychological well-being, which falls under the eudaimonic perspective, is thought to include six facets of actualization: mastery, life purpose, autonomy, self-acceptance, positive relationships, and personal growth.[6] Despite the different focus of these two perspectives, studies suggest that hedonic and eudaimonic well-being are often positively correlated and can even influence one another, indicating that they are overlapping yet distinct.[7]Further, individuals high in both hedonic and eudaimonic motives tend to experience the highest levels of overall well-being and are often considered to be thriving.[8]

Three Core Factors of Happiness

Various theories on happiness point to three core factors: *pleasure* (hedonism), *desire* (getting what you want), and *meaning* (living a purposeful life). These elements align with what psychologist Martin Seligman calls the *Authentic Happiness Theory.*[9]

---

3   Kahneman, 1999; Fredrickson, 2001.

4   Diener and Lucas, 1999; Diener, 2009.

5   Waterman, 1993; Ryff, 1995.

6   Ryff and Keyes, 1995.

7   King et al., 2006; Waterman, 2008; Huta and Ryan, 2010.

8   Huta and Ryan, 2010; Forgeard et al., 2011.

9   Seligman, 2003.

A 2019 meta-analysis by Joshua Ray Tanzer and Lisa Weyandt, using brain imaging to study happiness within Seligman's model, concluded that happiness is best understood not just as an affective state but as a byproduct of behavior and engagement. The authors explain, "For pleasure and engagement, this meant a literal relationship between behavioral and neurological activity. For meaning, this meant the ongoing assessment of the moral implications of events." [10]

Given the importance of pleasure, desire, and meaning in happiness, we can assume that the absence of pleasure, the presence of pain, a lack of ethical or moral values, and disengagement from meaningful goals can lead to a life that feels less fulfilling.

Moreover, an imbalance of these factors for happiness can lead to unhappiness. For instance, too much focus on pleasurable experiences without enough attention to meaningful goals can lead to emptiness. Likewise, focusing too much on desired outcomes without also seeking pleasure or meaning can result in unhappiness.

Behavioral Engagement: A Key to Lasting Happiness

Behavioral engagement is essential for genuine, lasting happiness. While simply daydreaming of pleasure, goals, or meaningful engagement can bring feelings of happiness, those sensations are typically short-lived without the kinetic and behavioral components needed to bring ideas to fruition. More often than not, these pursuits must be coupled with a sense of meaning beyond the quotidian and profane. We must activate this potential through practical, intentional actions directed toward our goals.

What Are We Running From?

As we traverse every nook and cranny of a mysterious, eerie, strange but beautiful world in the search for happiness, we must sometimes pause to

---

10   Tanzer and Weyandt, 2019.

assess the "why" of our every move and motive. From time immemorial, human beings have sought and found myriad creative ways to extend their experience of comfort and their sense of safety in what they *know* in order to avoid the inescapable uncertainty of the unknown and uncomfortable.

And why not?

After all, we live in a world pervaded by volatility, uncertainty, complexity, and ambiguity, the grandest of them being, as far as we know, the permanence of the greatest unknown, death. This programmed, gene-deep fear of death emerges from the abyss of the mind and body and manifests as an extemporized representation of the condition of our subconscious.

Our conditioning and programming, exhibited through the drama of our lives and the lives of others, have been woven into us by thousands of years of fear and the insatiable craving for safety. Our universe's Lovecraftian intelligence renders Earth's most brilliant minds obtuse, addled by ineptitude and bereft of the answer to one simple question: Why? This inquiry continues to plague us and, despite our industrial and technological innovations, brings us no closer to our need for existential closure.

As a species, we are the perpetual binky-faced toddler stuck in the developmental phase of the terrible twos, suddenly conscious in a seemingly alien planet and desperate for knowledge, agency, and autonomy, and yet cursed to be at the mercy of a stoic, dispassionate, inscrutable, and aesthetically grotesque universe in no hurry to explain or unveil itself.

False Consciousness

The term *false consciousness* refers to a distorted view that keeps people unaware of their own disadvantage. Rooted in Marxist theory, it originally described how oppressed groups can unknowingly accept beliefs and behaviors that work against their own best interests.

John T. Jost's definition provides a helpful starting point: "A consciousness is 'false' when it serves to perpetuate inequality by leading members of a subordinate group to believe that they are inferior, deserving of their plight, or incapable of taking action against the causes of their subordination."[11]

In other words, false consciousness can lead individuals to accept negative beliefs about themselves or their situations, reinforcing a cycle of limitation and unhappiness. When individuals hold false beliefs contrary to their well-being, they can unknowingly contribute to their own disadvantaged position and adopt a negative outlook on themselves, others, and the world around them. The psychological consequences of this phenomenon can be far-reaching, often preventing people from recognizing the need for change or collective action.

Now, we'll explore how false consciousness manifests in psychology and its connection to the illusion of happiness.

In psychology, false consciousness goes beyond politics; it includes mental patterns such as biases; defense mechanisms; the habitus that individuals, subgroups, and whole communities tend to adopt; and unconscious beliefs that shape our worldview. It can act as a psychological blind spot, leading individuals to unknowingly perpetuate emotions, beliefs, myths, and behaviors that reinforce their self-identity, even if that identity is based on misconceptions. This narrow perspective often arises from an unconscious desire to feel safe and avoid imaginary pain, similar to the concept of the panopticon.

The Panopticon of the Unconscious

The panopticon metaphor, popularized by philosopher Michel Foucault, describes a prison design in which a central watchtower allows one guard to observe all inmates while the inmates never know when they are being watched. The guard represents a "powerful other" whose ever-possible presence keeps the inmates obedient even though they cannot see him.

In the context of false consciousness, this concept takes on new meaning. Instead of a physical prison, individuals are often trapped within the limitations

---

11 Jost, 1995, p. 400.

of their own cognitive, behavioral, and emotional patterns, unable to recognize the internal and external influences that maintain their false consciousness. In this context, the "powerful other" isn't a literal authority figure but rather a kind of self-surveillance, a lens through which we monitor ourselves based on internalized beliefs and expectations. This hidden, self-imposed watcher keeps us bound to these beliefs, often as a result of a conditioned fear of the unknown. This influence operates beneath the surface, difficult to consciously identify, yet powerful in its ability to shape our decisions and outlook.

This psychological barrier keeps individuals entrenched in their unexamined beliefs, values, and behaviors, even when these are detrimental to their well-being. The obstacle manifests in countless ways: in distractions, in laziness, in fear, and in mundane activities that drain our vitality. By keeping our vision limited, this barrier misuses and disperses energy that could otherwise be directed toward change, growth, and other adaptive exploits.

The Illusion of Happiness

One significant consequence of false consciousness is the creation of an *illusion of happiness*. What is this illusion? It's a set of commodified beliefs and goals that we subscribe to, often unquestioningly, in the hope that participating in these socially prescribed rituals will lead to happiness.

This illusion takes shape as you pursue and then finally attain a supposedly valuable goal, only to realize that the excitement wears off after a few days, months, or years. It's a dream that society has advertised as a capital-T Truth without your full awareness. Many people recognize this feeling.

Think of how often we've been told that graduating from high school, going to college, finding a dream job, or meeting that soulmate will make us happy. Are these really *your* dreams? Or are they derivatives of stale dreams belonging to your family, your community, or even some larger institution?

These dreams and beliefs represent only a small part of the bill of goods we're all sold, and they go much deeper than this. Where do these thoughts come from? How did we swallow the bait, hook, line, and sinker?

False consciousness has profound psychological effects. It transmits to us an agitative dissonance that inevitably leads to emotional distress and illnesses of the body and mind instead of the dreams that once haloed our guileless heads.

Consider, for instance, someone who remains in a difficult relationship, convinced that the time, energy, and emotions they've invested are reason enough to stay. They may even go so far as convincing themselves they're happy to avoid confronting the painful truth of the situation. This is an example of a common logical fallacy called the *sunk cost fallacy*, in which a person is reluctant to change course because of how much they've already invested in their current situation, even when changing course would be the better option. These false beliefs perpetuate suffering and prevent adaptive change. In this case, the person may believe they need to stay in the relationship to feel valued or safe, even if it means staying in a cycle of dissatisfaction that, in the process called *homeostasis*, has become the norm for them.

Often we hold onto false beliefs or engage in ineffective behaviors because they provide us with a sense of security, even when those beliefs work against our true self-interest. False consciousness, when unexamined, doesn't lead to authentic well-being. Instead, it serves as a defense mechanism, shielding us from the discomfort that arises when we confront our vulnerability and uncertainty in relation to the world around us.

False Consciousness Is Holding You Back

False consciousness plays a role in our daily lives by subtly influencing us to maintain thoughts, beliefs, and behaviors that keep us stuck in old, decaying patterns. These patterns create a sense of stability, but they also trap us in a state of pseudo-happiness, an illusion of happiness that provides short-term comfort but ultimately hinders true personal growth.

This illusion may feel reassuring, but it prevents us from seeking genuine well-being. Recognizing and addressing our unique versions of false consciousness is essential for self-awareness, mental health, and, ultimately, the pursuit of happiness.

False consciousness often emerges from deeply ingrained, subconscious beliefs and behaviors that we have been prescribed or we've adopted to protect ourselves from emotional pain. These beliefs are powerful—they form self-limiting myths, emotions, and actions that prevent growth. But until we are aware of and can recognize this false consciousness, we can't identify how or where it's holding us back. Here are some common ways false consciousness traps us:

- **Maintaining the Status Quo:** False consciousness perpetuates the status quo, even when it's harmful. Many people hold on to destructive habits, toxic relationships, or unfulfilling jobs because they have been convinced that these situations bring happiness. In reality, they're caught in a cycle of conformity to social norms and expectations, unable to break free.

- **Resistance to Change:** False consciousness fosters resistance to change by reinforcing the belief that any deviation from the familiar will lead to unhappiness or anxiety-producing situations. Fear of such outcomes can manifest as a reluctance to pursue passions, explore new paths, or embrace personal growth.

- **Cognitive Dissonance:** Living with false consciousness often leads to cognitive dissonance; the tension and discomfort that arise when our values, beliefs, and actions don't align. This internal conflict can create anxiety, depression, and a pervasive sense of unease, making it hard to take calculated risks in order to attain authentic happiness.

As you can see, the illusion of happiness is closely intertwined with false consciousness. This illusion gives us a façade of comfort, masking underlying dissatisfaction. It's easy to find temporary gratification in distractions, overindulgences (in food, for example), technology, or material comforts, but these fleeting moments of pleasure distract us from addressing the root causes of unhappiness.

Often, we avoid confronting painful realities such as unresolved trauma, unfulfilled dreams and visions, or dysfunctional relationships. This avoidance may temporarily preserve our comfort but ultimately prevents growth and self-discovery. Many of us chase superficial markers of happiness, social status, wealth, or external validation, rather than seeking genuine fulfillment. In the long term, this can lead to emptiness and a disconnect from our true selves.

Breaking the Illusion and Moving Forward

False consciousness and the illusion of happiness are powerful barriers to leading an authentically happy and flourishing life. Recognizing their influence and allure is the first step toward liberation. By cultivating self-awareness, embracing change, pursuing meaning and purpose, and building resilience, we can break free from these chains and embark on a journey of self-discovery. This journey leads to true, lasting contentment that comes from aligning with our real values and desires.

So, how do we begin this journey? In the next chapter, we'll explore the practical steps to confront false consciousness and break away from the illusions holding us back. Through these steps, you'll be equipped to start building a life aligned with your authentic self and uncover the path to genuine happiness.

Pause and Reflect

- Reflect on how often you engage in pleasurable experiences. Are these experiences aligned with your vision of your ideal self, or someone else's?
- Reflect on your mindset. If others could hear what you say about yourself, what would they think of you?
- Reflect on moments when you obtained a desire or reached a goal. What motivated you to do so?
- Reflect on experiences you've found meaningful. How often do you engage in meaningful experiences?
- List three times fear and procrastination prevented you from taking action towards achieving fulfillment in your life.
- Has your idea of happiness evolved as you have grown older, or has it remained the same since childhood?
- Identify one thing you can start doing, one thing you can continue doing, and one thing you can stop doing that will enhance your quality of life.

Prescribed Philosophies

We see through borrowed eyes. Much of what we believe to be our own perspective is an inheritance. The first step to seeing clearly is questioning who handed you the lens.

- Freedom is an unlearning process. Freedom and agency are about not just acquiring more knowledge but shedding illusions. What false narratives about yourself do you still hold onto?
- Comfort and happiness are not the same. You can be comfortable, but that will not necessarily make you feel fulfilled.
- Contentment comes not from accumulation but from alignment with your vision and values. Many people chase after material things, not realizing that having less would actually bring them closer to peace than having more.
- Happiness was defined for us before we could define it for ourselves. Have you ever stopped to ask if those definitions are truly yours?
- Happiness isn't outsourced. No person or achievement can fill an inner void. Where are you expecting the external to fix the internal?
- Happiness is uncovered, not acquired. Joy is already within you, buried under fears and false beliefs. What must you unlearn to access it?

CHAPTER 2.

HEART

"Clarity about what matters provides
clarity about what does not."[12]

—CAL NEWPORT

I n the previous chapter, we explored how false consciousness and the illusion of happiness can keep us stuck in cycles of self-deception, preventing us from leading an authentic, fulfilling life. When we become aware of the beliefs and behaviors that bind us, we open the door to a new kind of freedom: the freedom to redefine our lives and rewrite our stories based on values that resonate deeply with who we are.

But awareness alone, while essential, is only the beginning. True transformation requires an intentional, structured approach to reshape our daily lives and align our actions with our authentic selves. This is where HEART comes in. HEART offers a road map for building a life rooted in purpose, resilience, and

---

12   Cal Newport, Deep Work: Rules for Focused Success in a Distracted World, Grand Central Publishing, 2016.

genuine happiness. It guides us through a process of introspection, mindful engagement, and deliberate action, helping us to shed the layers of conditioning and illusion that have shaped our narratives up to this point.

The crux of this chapter is the framework of HEART and the five core facets of life it addresses: Health, Enterprise, Authentic Relationships, Recreation and Recovery, and Transcendent Purpose and Meaning. Each facet is an opportunity to bring our values, principles, beliefs, and personal philosophy into alignment, creating a foundation for a life that reflects our true selves.

With HEART, we don't aim to "fix" ourselves in pursuit of some perfect ideal. Instead, we build a system to foster resilience, self-awareness, and intentionality, cultivating a life worth living, one guided by our own aspirations and values. As we dive into this chapter, consider HEART your toolkit for transformation, supporting you in the journey toward authentic happiness and a more meaningful life.

HEART is a systems-based approach for engaging with both your inner and outer worlds, designed to help you achieve your vision while pursuing a life of true, lasting happiness—*eudaimonic happiness*. This framework doesn't rely on surface-level fixes; instead, it focuses on developing mindful awareness, which is essential for recognizing and addressing false consciousness and the illusions we may have built around our lives.

Key Strategies for Identifying Your HEART Priorities

Through the HEART concept, you'll be able to identify and break free from the self-limiting beliefs and habits that may be holding you back. Below are the key strategies you'll use to begin your journey:

- **Self-Awareness as the Foundation:** Overcoming false consciousness begins with self-awareness. By reflecting deeply on your beliefs, values, and behaviors, you can identify areas where you may be limiting yourself. This process can be aided through therapy, counseling, mentorship, or introspective practices such as mindfulness meditation.

- **Embracing Change and Growth:** Living authentically means welcoming change as a pathway to growth and self-discovery. This often involves stepping out of your comfort zone and confronting fears. Seeking guidance from a mentor, therapist or coach can provide invaluable support throughout this transformative journey.

- **Pursuing Transcendent Purpose and Eudaimonic Happiness:** True happiness arises from a sense of purpose and meaning. Instead of chasing fleeting pleasures, HEART encourages exploring your passions and values and aligning your actions with your authentic self.

- **Building Resilience and Antifragility:** Breaking free from entrenched patterns can be challenging, which is why resilience and antifragility are key elements of this system. Antifragility, the ability to grow stronger through adversity, and emotional resilience are crucial for managing the discomfort and uncertainty that often accompany self-discovery. Action, mindfulness routines, an adaptive mindset, social support, and self-care are essential in this process.

The Five Facets of HEART

HEART is designed to guide you in making real, impactful changes across five key areas of life: Health, Enterprise, Authentic Relationships, Recreation and Recovery, and Transcendent Purpose. Each of these facets is essential to living a balanced and meaningful life and encourages you to think deeply about how your values, principles, ideals, beliefs, and personal philosophy connect to each one. Through this approach, you'll develop your own path to a life of eudaimonic happiness, a life genuinely worth living.

Here's how each facet contributes to the framework:

- **Health** encompasses physical, mental, emotional, and spiritual well-being. It's more than the absence of illness or discomfort; it includes the presence of positive factors that enhance vitality and quality of life. Reflecting on health through HEART means exploring how your values guide your approach to wellness—prioritizing self-care, balance, and growth to create a foundation for overall happiness.

- **Enterprise** refers to the pursuit of meaningful work or learning that enables you to maintain a chosen lifestyle. This facet includes the pursuit of career goals, financial security, and the development of skills and personal growth within a chosen field or industry. Enterprise is about securing resources for sustenance, security, and personal fulfillment. Using HEART, you'll examine the beliefs and ideals that shape your professional life and consider whether you could better align your work with your values to create a career that's more rewarding, fulfilling and meaningful.

- **Authentic Relationships** are the connections we maintain with ourselves and others, such as family, friends, romantic partners, colleagues, our community, and even nature. Healthy relationships are built on trust, mutual respect, connectedness, and reciprocity, all of which contribute to emotional well-being and a sense of belonging. HEART encourages you to consider the ideals and principles that guide your interactions so you can nurture relationships that align with your authentic self and support your journey.

- **Recreation and Recovery** is the process of restoring physical, mental, and emotional well-being after experiencing challenges, setbacks, or stress. It involves deliberate efforts to rejuvenate and heal through rest, relaxation, play, and self-care. Recreation and Recovery also includes engaging in creative outlets that promote mental flexibility and refresh the mind. HEART invites you to look at how your values and beliefs support recreation and to prioritize restorative activities that foster resilience and a well-rounded life.

- **Transcendent Purpose and Meaning** refers to a profound sense of purpose, meaning and fulfillment. This stance requires every moment to be viewed as important. Transcendence is more than mere existence or living life on autopilot. It's about pursuing passions and visions that provide a sense of significance. Meaning comes from the narrative you create throughout your journey, the story you want to tell and that you want others to remember. In HEART, purpose connects deeply to the drive that reinforces your personal philosophy, embodying your highest values and ideals to guide you toward a life of enduring happiness and contentment.

Connect These Key Concepts

To get your HEART journey underway, it's essential to reflect on how each of the Five Facets connects to core inner concepts: *values, principles, ideals, beliefs,* and *personal philosophy.* Recognizing and understanding these terms will help you build a solid foundation for living an authentic, meaningful life aligned with your true self.

- **Values** are deeply held beliefs about what is important and desirable in life. Acting as our moral compass, values guide our decisions, actions, and priorities, shaping our ethical choices and forming the basis for personal and societal norms.
- **Principles** are fundamental guidelines that govern behavior and decisions, derived from our core values. Self-adopted principles translate values into actionable rules, creating consistency in how we make choices and interact with the world.
- **Ideals** are visionary standards of excellence that we aspire to but may find challenging to fully achieve. They represent our highest hopes and goals, motivating us toward improvement, personal growth, and societal progress.
- **Beliefs** are convictions or assumptions about the truth or existence of something, often rooted in personal experience, faith, or evidence. These beliefs shape our worldview, influencing our values, principles, and behaviors, and coloring how we perceive reality.
- **Personal philosophy** is a structured framework of thought that explores reality, ethics, and existence. Our personal philosophy encompasses values, principles, ideals, and beliefs, offering a coherent perspective through which we understand ourselves and the world. It's a lens that helps us build self-awareness, guiding us toward a meaningful, intentional life.

While these five concepts share commonalities, each plays a distinct role in shaping thought, behavior, and the pursuit of understanding:

- **Hierarchy:** At the foundation, values drive our principles. Principles translate values into action, while ideals represent our highest aspirations. Beliefs shape how we perceive reality, and our personal philosophy ties all these elements together, providing structure and depth.

- **Specificity:** Values and principles tend to be more specific and concrete, guiding daily choices and ethics, while ideals are more abstract, embodying our loftiest aspirations. Beliefs vary widely, covering everything from personal convictions to religious doctrines, while philosophy takes a broader, systematic view of these elements.

- **Flexibility:** Beliefs may evolve as we gain new experiences and insights, while principles, though rooted in values, can adapt to different situations. Ideals are often long-term but may shift as circumstances change. Values and philosophy are more enduring, offering stable foundations over time.

Understanding these distinctions will reward you with a deeper appreciation for the complexity and richness of the human experience and how it influences your worldview, behavior, and choices.

It's important, however, to ask yourself whether the values, principles, beliefs, and philosophies you hold truly belong to you or whether they've been influenced by powerful forces such as family, religion, culture, zeitgeist, epoch, media, or institutions. Through introspection and rigorous self-examination, you can distinguish between what is genuinely yours and what you may have been conditioned to believe by others.

Breaking Free from False Consciousness

False consciousness reveals how individuals can unknowingly adopt beliefs and behaviors that reinforce their own unhappiness. Much like inmates in a panopticon, they are monitored by an unseen, powerful force, often their own subconscious fears and uncertainties, keeping them trapped in a cycle of fear and self-limitation. The illusion of happiness, closely tied to false consciousness, masks underlying dissatisfaction with fleeting gratifications, preventing individuals from fully acknowledging their own nature, desires, and needs.

Together, false consciousness and the illusion of happiness create a powerful barrier that keeps people bound to the status quo, resistant to change, and burdened by cognitive dissonance. The illusion provides temporary comfort, allowing us to sidestep uncomfortable truths and live behind a façade of contentment. However, as we've explored, this comfort is only a shadow of the authentic happiness that comes from living with purpose, intention, and alignment with our values, principles, and beliefs.

So how can one truly break free from false consciousness? Here are some steps to help you:

1. **Cultivate self-awareness and a desire for discovery.** On the journey to true happiness, self-awareness acts as a guiding light, helping us navigate out of the shadows of false consciousness. By carefully examining our values, principles, ideals, beliefs, and philosophical foundations, we begin to peel back the layers of conditioning, self-deception, and avoidance that keep us entangled in the patterns of our current lives. This is the first step in our journey to enjoying a truly fulfilling life.

2. **Summon your courage and be willing to face discomfort.** The shallow gratifications we often chase must give way to the deeper, enduring fulfillment that emerges when we live in alignment with our core values and principles. We must be willing to confront painful truths and embrace the transformative potential of change.

3. **Learn the power of letting go and embracing change.** Change is inevitable and a constant in life. Shedding outdated belief systems frees us to form a worldview that aligns with our evolving understanding. Some of the most defining moments of our lives occur when we stop resisting change and instead lean into it. True liberation is found not in rigid certainty but in the flexibility to evolve.

By following the steps above, you can uncover the essence of a life truly worth living, one marked by authenticity, purpose, and a renewed sense of aliveness. Authenticity doesn't require perfection; rather, it calls for a commitment to change, flexibility, self-discovery, and personal growth. Genuine happiness, you'll realize, is not a fleeting emotion but a steady state of being, rooted in living a life that is true to yourself.

In the next chapter, we will discuss the why of HEART; dive deeper into how your values, principles, ideals, beliefs, and philosophy relate directly to your HEART; and talk about how to begin building the scaffold that will become your pathway to success. Before you head to Chapter 3, be sure to complete the reflection exercise below; it will help put you in the right mindset for this journey.

Pause and Reflect

Some reflection questions to get you started on your HEART journey:

- Recall moments when you felt genuinely happy and content. What were the circumstances, and what made those moments special?
- What has been your personal experience of false consciousness? Have there been moments when you realized that you were pursuing an illusion of happiness? What were the consequences, and how did you address them?
- Have you ever found yourself holding onto beliefs or behaviors that seemed to bring comfort but were ultimately detrimental to your well-being in the long run? List three such occasions.
- How do you generally respond to challenges in your life? Do you tend to avoid them, or do you confront them head-on?
- How do you typically respond to change in your life? Do you resist it, embrace it, or something in between? Has change at times caused you unpleasant and ineffective thoughts, behaviors, and emotions? If so, list three such times.
- Consider the definition of success you've been conditioned to believe. Where did it come from: family, culture, society? Does this definition truly resonate with you? If not, how would you redefine success in a way that aligns with your deepest values and aspirations?

- Think about a major goal or aspiration you've been pursuing. What is the deeper motivation behind it? Is it driven by a genuine desire, a need for external validation, or a fear of failure? If you removed external pressures and expectations, would this still be something you truly want?

Prescribed Philosophies

- Prioritization of health is a lifestyle as important as eating, drinking water, and breathing. The degree to which you prioritize your health can determine the quality of your human experience.
- Your community of origin is not the arbiter of truth.
- Implementing consistency, routines, and adaptive systems of thought, feeling, and behavior will set you apart from most people.
- Filtering out the necessary from the unnecessary will change your life.
- Generational trauma is real. So are generational blessings. Be the ancestor your descendants will be thankful for.
- Many of the dysfunctions you see in your culture, community, family, and self today are rooted in history and society. Be careful when you point blame.
- Most of your fears are nothing but shadows and illusions. Letting go of attachments to external sources of validation allows us to put our fears to rest and build confidence from within.

CHAPTER 3.

Why Does HEART Work?

"The Second Law [of Thermodynamics] defines the ultimate purpose of life, mind, and human striving: to deploy energy and information to fight back the tide of entropy and carve out refuges of beneficial order."[13]

—STEVEN PINKER

I n Chapter 2, we explored the concept of HEART, a framework for building a life of purpose that's aligned with your core values. As you begin using HEART to discover the deep contentment that comes from living authentically, you may wonder why this approach is so essential. In this chapter, we will look at the "why" behind HEART, examining the reasons a life structured around authenticity and eudaimonic happiness can create lasting fulfillment.

Your values, principles, ideals, beliefs, and philosophy aren't just abstract ideas, they are the building blocks that make up the framework of a life worth

---

13   Steven Pinker, "The Second Law of Thermodynamics," Edge.org, 2017, https://www.edge.org/response-detail/27023/.

living. Here, we'll connect these core aspects of your identity to a practical structure that will guide you toward fulfillment. Think of this chapter as a bridge, linking your current understanding with the steps you'll take to build the life you envision. Together, we'll begin constructing the framework that can serve as your pathway to lasting happiness. Let's get started!

Negentropy—How We Counteract Entropy

Despite our efforts to attain peace and harmony in life, we often encounter dissatisfaction, unmet expectations, and disappointment. In trying to fill this inner void, we can fall into cognitive, behavioral, and emotional patterns that ultimately increase feelings of chaos and disorder. This sense of inner turmoil is a psychological state of entropy, where our inner and outer worlds seem to devolve into confusion, exhaustion, unpredictability, and disarray.

In Chapter 2, we explored the challenges of living in a VUCA world (volatile, uncertain, complex, and ambiguous). These unpredictable conditions often leave us feeling apprehensive about making choices, leading to a persistent sense of insecurity.

Shattered Assumptions Theory, introduced by Ronnie Janoff-Bulman, suggests that we all hold core beliefs about the world, others, and ourselves, beliefs that serve as the foundation for how we navigate life. For example, one might believe that the world is benevolent (generally safe and just), that the world is meaningful (has order and purpose), and that one is worthy (deserves love and respect). When trauma or significant disruption occurs, these assumptions can be shattered, forcing the person to confront the uncomfortable truth that the world may not be as safe, purposeful, or fair as once believed.

Many of the most volatile, unpredictable situations we encounter stem from areas of life that are fundamental to our well-being: our health, relationships, resources (such as financial stability or education), our capacity for adaptive coping and creativity, and our sense of purpose. The erosion of any of these pillars can leave us feeling unmoored. Chronic stress, illness, or neglecting self-care amplifies our sense of disorder, while uncertainty in relationships, due to communication breakdowns, fear of rejection, or shifting dynamics, can lead to emotional isolation and dysregulation. Additionally, the pressure to secure resources and maintain stability can foster a deep sense of powerlessness. Without regular moments of play, creativity, and rest, we become trapped in cycles of exhaustion, depleting our capacity for joy and rejuvenation. Most profoundly, a loss of purpose can leave us adrift, disengaged, and vulnerable to despair.

When any of these areas fall into disorder, the imbalance cascades, affecting every part of our lives and shattering the assumptions we once held about ourselves and the world. Healing requires rebuilding these assumptions, a process that involves not just recovering but evolving and aligning more deeply with our values.

This is where HEART comes in. HEART provides a base from which to operate, a ballast that helps us counteract the external forces that relentlessly test our resolve. By restoring balance and offering clarity, HEART helps us navigate the complexities of life with greater resilience. This concept of balance aligns with the principle of *negentropy*, an adaptive response that restores order and flow in the midst of chaos. HEART is a *negentropic* approach that counteracts the entropy of modern life. At its core, HEART connects our deepest values, beliefs, and ideals, guiding us toward a more purposeful, fulfilling life. In this way, HEART becomes a tool not only for healing but for rebuilding the assumptions that trauma or disruption have shaken, helping us forge a new path forward.

How does HEART accomplish this?

- **Clarifying Values:** Before constructing your HEART, you must begin a journey of deep self-reflection. This process isn't just about listing values but about understanding why they matter to you. HEART prompts you to explore the core priorities and principles that guide your decisions and actions. It encourages you to identify values that resonate most deeply with your true self.
- **Aligning with Purpose:** Once your values are clear, HEART helps you align them with your overarching purpose. It's not enough to hold values; they must be directed toward a clear and meaningful goal. HEART

ensures that your values become a compass, guiding you toward a life that reflects what genuinely matters to you.

- **Navigating External Chaos:** In our VUCA world, external factors can easily throw even the most grounded individuals off balance. However, a life guided by HEART is more resilient in the face of such forces. By integrating your purpose and values into your daily decisions and actions, you build a strong internal framework. This framework acts as a stabilizing force, enabling you to weather life's storms with a sense of direction and purpose.
- **Recognizing Assumptions:** Understanding and acknowledging our core assumptions about the world, ourselves, and others is crucial because these beliefs shape our perceptions, decisions, and responses to challenges. By recognizing these assumptions, we can identify whether they are based on outdated or distorted experiences that affect our HEART priorities, opening the door to growth, adaptation, and healthier coping strategies in the face of life's uncertainties.

As you construct your HEART priorities and weave together your purpose, values, principles, ideals, beliefs, and philosophy, you create a reservoir of strength and clarity. This reservoir becomes your anchor, providing stability and resilience in a world where everything can shift in an instant. Embracing HEART allows you to chart a course toward a life worth living and to find balance in the turmoil, anchoring your life in authenticity, vision, and purpose.

Self-Reflection Is Tough but Vital

In our journey toward fulfillment and genuine happiness, HEART serves as a guiding beacon, granting us the power to shape the life we desire. However, it's essential to recognize that no matter which path we choose, we will inevitably encounter pain and challenges that test our strength. The lives of those we admire, whether in our own circles or in the broader context of history, possess a common thread: these people faced and overcame obstacles on their way to purpose and fulfillment.

Consider the life of Nelson Mandela, a global symbol of resilience and unwavering dedication to justice. Mandela's journey involved enduring immense hardship, including spending twenty-seven years in prison for his activism against apartheid in South Africa. Throughout those years, his commitment to equality and freedom remained unshaken. Mandela's sacrifices ultimately helped dismantle an oppressive system and paved the way for reconciliation and democracy in South Africa.

Similarly, Marie Curie, the pioneering scientist, made extraordinary sacrifices in her relentless pursuit of scientific discovery. Her groundbreaking research on radiation, which came at the cost of her health, laid the foundation for significant advancements in science and medicine.

These stories remind us that greatness often arises from a willingness to embrace the challenges and sacrifices required to lead a life worth living. The sacrifices these individuals made were investments in a future they believed in, a future that transcended personal comfort for the greater good. This book advocates for choosing a life that is worth the challenges it presents, recognizing that sacrifices are both necessary and meaningful.

HEART empowers you to embark on your own journey with values, principles, and purpose. It's a compass that guides you through life's inevitable challenges. HEART serves as a framework not only for navigating life but also for embracing the meaningful sacrifices necessary to live a life of authenticity and fulfillment.

Building a Balanced Life with HEART

The purpose of HEART is to provide direction in life, a quality many of us seek but often find elusive. Life's complexities can feel overwhelming; just as one problem is solved, another seems to emerge out of nowhere.

HEART offers a way to organize this overwhelming world into manageable parts, helping us create a structure that brings clarity and purpose to our lives. HEART does this by focusing on five distinct areas: Health, Enterprise, Authentic Relationships, Recreation and Recovery, and Transcendent Purpose and Meaning. These areas correspond to our fundamental needs and form the foundation for a well-rounded, intentional life.

By dividing life into these five areas, HEART allows us to focus on each one thoughtfully. Together, these areas create a scaffold that grounds our values and provides a practical way to organize life around what truly matters.

As you work with HEART, consider the role of five processes: Time, Resistance, Change, Control, and Awareness (TRACE). These processes shape our lives depending on how effectively we engage with them. How we choose to spend our time, for example, profoundly affects our growth, while awareness, our ability to learn and to understand ourselves and our surroundings, determines our capacity for intentional decision-making. These constants form a framework within HEART itself, offering a deeper level of agency over our choices and actions.

Once your HEART is outlined, the next step is to assess the skills and capabilities needed to live according to your chosen values. This isn't just about acquiring new skills; it's about embodying your values through consistent action. As you align your actions with your principles, you begin to experience the strength and integrity that come from living authentically.

With HEART as your foundation, achievements that may have once seemed distant begin to feel within reach, and the life you envision starts to take shape. HEART offers a structure that brings balance and intentionality to life, setting you on a path toward enduring happiness.

Throughout this book, we'll continue exploring what it means to create a life worth living, including the actionable steps that can bring you closer to that vision. Your HEART will serve as a guide, helping you choose a mission that aligns with your values and moves you toward a purposeful life.

To thrive, you need vitality in both body and mind. To conceptualize the importance of HEART, imagine trying to survive in a jungle. Just as surviving in nature requires energy, strategy, and resilience, navigating life's complexities demands physical well-being, mental flexibility, and awareness of the world around you. This means discerning what truly matters versus what distracts you, and identifying habits or influences that help or hinder your growth.

In the wild, survival is about more than just foraging and hunting; it's about reading the environment—shifts in weather, changes in animal behavior, and ecosystemic patterns—all of which shape your ability to thrive. These elements form your survival toolkit.

In an unpredictable world, thriving isn't something you do alone. True fulfillment and resilience come from building authentic connections, starting with yourself, then extending to others and even to the natural world around you. The contributions you make to your social circle, whether those contributions are big or small, shape your role in it and impact the strength of your support system. In this dance of survival, you're not just a passive participant; you're an essential contributor. Your unique strengths, insights, and connections define your role and the quality of your experience.

Amid the demands of living with intention, moments of rest, play, and introspection become vital. These pauses are where creativity, flexibility, and innovation emerge, helping us stay open, grounded, and rejuvenated in our purpose. Above all, a life worth living requires a transcendent sense of purpose and meaning, a narrative or story beyond the mundane, the driving force that sustains us through challenges and motivates us to keep moving forward even when circumstances feel uncertain.

Without a clear understanding of what constitutes a life worth living, many of us find ourselves trapped in a disheartening cycle of ennui. This prevailing listlessness casts a pall over our lives, a dullness that persists from the moment we wake until nightfall. Even then, the perseverating thoughts continue. The lack of excitement and vibrancy in each passing day reflects a more profound discontent that gnaws at our very essence. In the search for any kind of excitement to quell this dissatisfaction, we often turn to activities that serve as temporary distractions from the underlying sense that something crucial is amiss. What we need isn't yet another distraction but rather an urgent investigation, an excavation to unearth the root causes of this pervasive dissatisfaction and disconnection from our sense of meaning and what truly matters. Only then can we break the cycle.

The disconnect is everywhere. It's in how you see yourself versus how others see you. It's in the shallow distractions we call leisure and the nagging feeling that you're missing something vital. You feel adrift, detached from the purpose and the vibrant life you suspect you're meant to live.

I know that feeling; it's frustrating, exhausting, and easy to ignore, until you can no longer ignore it. But to move forward, you have to ask yourself the hard questions: What do you genuinely want? What do you truly need? It's not enough to chase fleeting desires and temporary pleasures. You need to sit with these questions, wrestle with them, and get real about your answers because the life you want starts with knowing what's worth wanting.

By using HEART, you learn to distinguish between fleeting desires and true needs. Have you taken the time to examine whether your pursuits reflect your core values? Do your daily actions support a meaningful life, or are they simply habits that have gone unquestioned?

HEART provides the tools to peel back the layers of conditioning and societal influence, helping you discover who you are at your core. This process of self-examination allows you to separate your authentic self from external expectations, building a foundation of integrity and authenticity. HEART will help you craft a life that minimizes regret, embraces adaptability, and evolves with you, reflecting both the person you are and the person you're becoming.

Bridging HEART to Action with TRACE

In the next chapter, we'll explore TRACE as an essential tool in your journey. You'll learn how each element of TRACE supports your HEART, amplifying your ability to pursue meaningful goals with resilience and adaptability. Together, HEART and TRACE create a comprehensive approach to living intentionally, balancing purpose with action and vision with progress.

As you complete this chapter, take a few moments to reflect on what you've uncovered so far. Your HEART principles will be the foundation of a life that aligns with your authentic self. Now, TRACE will serve as your road map, guiding you in translating this vision into achievable steps. Embrace this transition to the next chapter as a pivotal step toward a life worth living, one intentional, purposeful action at a time.

Pause and Reflect

Some reflection questions to help you on your HEART journey:

- Do your relationships reflect the value and resource quotient you bring to the group, as discussed in the chapter? How can you contribute more meaningfully to your social circles?
- How comfortable are you with uncertainty and evolving? Rank your comfort level from 1 to 5, with 5 being the most comfortable. What fears are keeping you from increasing your scores from a lower to a higher number?
- Have you ever pursued desires that ultimately left you unfulfilled? What were they? What lessons did you learn from that experience?
- Reflect on the concept of "fear of missing out" (FOMO) and its impact on your life. Is there a particular instance where participating in an activity you thought you were missing out on left you feeling empty?
- Using HEART as a guide, are there areas of your life where you feel an imbalance? List three examples from each priority (Health, Enterprise, Authentic Relationships, Recreation and Recovery, and Transcendent Purpose and Meaning).
- How has procrastination or avoidance played a role in costing you opportunities for growth in HEART?
- How do you plan on realigning your energy into your priorities this week?

Prescribed Philosophies

- The more complex our lives become, the more entropy we invite. Simplifying our thoughts, actions, and environments helps us navigate challenges with resilience, reducing disorder and enhancing our capacity for peace.
- Setting boundaries is an essential aspect of negentropy. By knowing where to draw lines in our time, energy, and commitments, we preserve our focus, reduce overwhelm, and create the space for meaningful engagement.
- Balance is the negentropic force. In the face of external volatility, we must maintain internal balance. By continuously realigning our priorities and energy, we can stabilize ourselves and create coherence in an otherwise unpredictable world.
- When faced with complexity, seek clarity through mindful reflection. By honing our awareness, we cut through the noise, allowing us to create a sense of calm amidst the chaos.
- Embrace challenges as opportunities to learn about yourself, your expectations, and your environment.
- Transformation isn't found in grand gestures but in the small moments of daily alignment of mind, body, and soul.
- Learning new skills can be challenging in the beginning. With practice, these new skills become second nature.

CHAPTER 4

Introducing TRACE— A Process for Fulfillment

"You do not rise to the level of your goals. You fall to the level of your systems."[14]

—JAMES CLEAR

A s you explore the HEART framework, you're establishing a foundation rooted in your values, principles, and goals, providing structure and purpose to your life. Constructing your HEART sets the stage for a life filled with intention and meaning. However, life's complexities require more than foundational principles alone; they require a method for setting and achieving goals aligned with those values. This is where the TRACE system comes in.

---

14 James Clear, "You do not rise [. . .]" (web page), jamesclear.com, https://jamesclear.com/quotes/you-do-not-rise-to-the-level-of-your-goals-you-fall-to-the-level-of-your-systems/.

TRACE—Time, Resistance, Awareness, Control, and Evolving—is a systemized process for unlocking potential and reaching milestones within the framework of your values, helping you stay on course as you navigate toward your vision. Just as HEART provides the foundation for a life worth living, TRACE offers a structured process to transform aspirations into tangible progress.

HEART defines what matters most to you, while TRACE equips you with the tools to stay resilient, make thoughtful decisions, and drive intentional change. Together, they form a cohesive framework, empowering you to live a life guided by clarity, intention, and purpose.

In this chapter, we'll break down each component of TRACE, exploring its role and showing how it integrates with the principles you've laid out in HEART. By the end of this chapter, you'll be ready to apply TRACE within the context of your HEART priorities, harnessing this framework to achieve authentic fulfillment and lasting success.

TRACE: Breaking Down the Acronym

TRACE is a method for navigating goals and growth, built on five essential components: Time, Resistance, Awareness, Control, and Evolving. Each element serves as a guide to achieving your vision while staying aligned with your priorities. More than a framework, TRACE is a continuous, ever-unfolding process, one we are always in the midst of, whether we recognize it or not. Time moves forward with or without our consent. Resistance challenges our growth. Awareness sharpens or fades. Control shifts between effort and surrender. And Evolving is inevitable, shaped by our responses at every turn. There is no point of stillness within TRACE, only movement, adaptation, and refinement. It is not a linear path with a one destination but rather a living, cyclical process that mirrors the rhythm of life itself. The question is not whether we are in it, but whether we are engaging with it intentionally. Let's explore each element and its role in shaping a life of meaning and purpose.

Time

Time, like an unceasing river, shapes our experiences and molds our future as it flows through our lives. Within the HEART framework, time becomes either the bedrock supporting our aspirations or the quicksand undermining them, depending on the care and intention with which you have invested your time. Some questions to consider include how you conceptualize time and how your goals and aspirations need both quality and quantity of time to grow and reach fruition.

For example, if you decide to dedicate time each week to your health, you might set aside hours for exercise, preparing nutritious meals, and finding moments for mental rejuvenation. But time isn't only about quantity; the quality of those hours is also crucial. If the hours you spend at the gym are full of distractions, for example, your progress may stall. By focusing on the quality of time you invest in each area, whether it's in authentic relationships, enterprise, recreation, or health, you open the door to deeper, more fulfilling progress.

A New Way of Looking at Time

When you think about time, especially of the past, what comes to mind? You might imagine those old, sepia-toned photographs or black-and-white films from a different era, reminders of lives lived in what feels like a distant past. But what if we shifted our perspective? Without the concept of calendars or clocks, the notion of time loses much of its structure, leaving us with only *now*. This present moment is, in fact, all we ever truly experience. Every event, from the past and into the future, unfolds within this eternal moment.

The time you have right now is your personal slice of eternity. Every choice you make, each action you take, and all your experiences are bound to this moment. This time is an irreplaceable resource. How you invest it, how you direct your energy and attention at this moment, becomes part of your legacy. The same moment that you experience now will connect you to future generations, much as it links you to those who came before.

Small-t time vs. capital-T Time

Think of your lifetime as small-t time—the time you have, the moments you live day to day. Capital-T Time is different: it is the vast, unchanging expanse of existence, encompassing the eons before and after you. Your life is but a drop of time in this endless ocean of time, a brief moment within an eternal moment. By mastering these two dimensions of time, you can live a life of transcendent purpose, one defined by meaningful action and lasting impact rather than missed opportunities and regret. So, how will you use your time in this eternal present? Do it now? Do it later? Whether you do or you don't, you're doing, you did, and you're done.

Resistance

Resistance is a natural part of any meaningful journey, challenging us in both internal and external ways. Within the TRACE framework, we distinguish two types of resistance: the internal, small-r resistance, representing doubts, fears, and personal tendencies; and the external, capital-R Resistance, encompassing societal pressures, obligations, and unforeseen challenges beyond our control.

Resistance can be either a barrier or a bridge to achieving your goals. It can be helpful or harmful. Resistance can show up as steadfastness, curiosity, or courage in the face of fear and challenges, or as avoidance, procrastination, excuses, or hesitation despite clear evidence in favor of action.

Within the HEART framework, being mindful of resistance, whether it's the quiet voice of self-doubt or the weight of external obstacles, is essential for growth. Consider the professional striving for a promotion or career change. Internal fears, compounded by external pressures such as societal expectations or competition, can feel overwhelming. However, by recognizing and anticipating these resistances, the person can prepare to navigate and overcome these hurdles.

When approached with awareness, resistance becomes adaptive: a catalyst for resilience and growth. By transforming resistance into motivation, you can strengthen your resolve and progress with purpose, aligning your efforts with what truly matters to you.

In the grand tapestry of life, resistance is a constant companion, often standing as a barrier between us and our aspirations. Yet, resistance also holds the potential to be a bridge, transforming obstacles into opportunities for growth. To navigate the labyrinthine paths of the HEART framework, we must first understand resistance's pervasive and dual nature.

Resistance as a Tool for Growth

When harnessed adaptively, resistance becomes a force for resilience. Adaptive resistance involves opposing harmful tendencies, such as negative thinking or destructive habits, that hinder progress. For example, resisting the impulse to procrastinate or indulge in self-sabotage strengthens resolve and promotes growth. Conversely, maladaptive resistance, like avoiding change or growth, leads to stagnation, often accompanied by feelings of regret, malaise, and missed opportunities.

Cultivating Robustness Through Resistance

Key qualities such as courage, grit, and antifragility are indispensable for transforming resistance into growth. In Nassim Nicholas Taleb's book *Antifragile: Things That Gain from Disorder* (2012), he uses his concept of antifragility to highlight how stressors can strengthen a system, preparing it to face future challenges more effectively. Similarly, grit and courage enable us to persevere through setbacks, fostering adaptability and long-term success.

Recognizing Resistance in Action

Consider an individual striving to improve their health. External resistance might take the form of demanding schedules or financial constraints, while internal resistance manifests as excuses, self-doubt, or fear of change. Awareness of these forces is the first step toward overcoming them. By developing adaptive strategies, such as prioritizing health within available resources and cultivating discipline, the individual paves the way to a healthier, more intentional life.

Regarding Enterprise, academic, professional, and financial success brings external challenges, such as workplace dynamics or uncertainty, while internal barriers like impostor syndrome, procrastination, laziness, or fear of failure can cast long shadows of regret and even more unforeseen consequences. Recognizing and addressing these resistances empowers individuals to climb the career ladder, build resilience, and restore financial stability.

In Authentic Relationships, resistance often reveals itself in reluctance to accept uncomfortable truths within our connections to family, friends, or partners. Maladaptive resistance can perpetuate unhealthy narratives and emotional stagnation. Resistance can keep us from deep connections with others and the natural world. Though it is sometimes painful to confront this resistance, doing so opens pathways to deeper understanding and authentic growth.

Resistance in this sphere of recreation and recovery may arise from societal expectations to stay perpetually productive or from internal struggles with discipline and motivation. By intentionally creating space for leisure and recovery, one can reclaim balance and explore creative outlets that rejuvenate the mind and spirit.

Pursuing a transcendent purpose often entails confronting external resistance, such as societal norms that discourage unconventional paths, and internal resistance, such as self-doubt, ignorance, procrastination, comfort, and laziness. By understanding the roots of these challenges and strategically addressing them, individuals become advocates for their cause, grounded in their values.

The Shadow of Resistance

Unchecked resistance casts a shadow over our lives, manifesting as inertia, quiet desperation, envy, or regret. This shadow reminds us of opportunities squandered due to fear, lack of information, or inaction. Yet, by confronting resistance head-on, we illuminate a path toward growth and enlightenment.

Across the HEART framework, the omnipresence of resistance underscores the importance of self-awareness and deliberate planning. By identifying and addressing internal and external sources of resistance, we build fortitude, align with our values, and move closer to the life we envision.

Awareness

Awareness is focused on expanding our understanding of the actions, emotions, and thoughts of ourselves and others while being attuned to the worlds within and around us. Within TRACE, awareness complements HEART by honing focus and clarity, filtering information, and revealing situational and life patterns, phases, cycles, and blind spots that may impact your goals.

Self-awareness also lets you reflect on how well your actions align with your values, creating more mindful engagement in each important aspect of your life. It empowers you to make informed decisions and adapt your strategies as needed.

As we take our turns on the floor in this *danse macabre* called life, awareness serves as a floodlight, illuminating our path as we seek solid footing amidst the challenge of staying aligned with our TRACE processes and HEART priorities. When harnessed effectively, these twin forces empower us to make conscious, informed decisions that shape the landscapes of our existence. Awareness encompasses not only our internal and external experiences, beliefs, thoughts, and assumptions but also our capacity for attention, filtering, focus, concentration, and wisdom, constantly evolving through more experience, knowledge, and learning. Awareness allows us to look beyond surface reactions and explore the underlying patterns and beliefs that influence our experiences.

Poor self-awareness can lead to myriad issues. Lack of awareness renders your priorities vulnerable to undesirable elements. You may manage to stumble through life, but it's like feeling your way in the dark, going astray as you search for objects that can be found only with light. Now imagine how far you could go if you weren't just illuminated but also deeply attuned to what you were searching for. Poor self-awareness inevitably leads to unnecessary pain and suffering. Yet, do not despair, luck may occasionally intervene. After all, even a broken clock is right twice a day.

Still, life is already rife with inevitable misfortunes. To compound these with avoidable ignorance is nothing short of a Shakespearean tragedy. When we lack internal and external awareness, we are unable to interpret our own experience meaningfully and accurately.

In this state, we neither reflect on nor question our beliefs, thoughts, emotions, and behaviors. We rarely pause to ask why we hold our views or react in specific ways. We fail to interrogate our ontological stance or our glib responses to the monotonous trivialities we mistake for sustenance or depth. Instead, we drift through life preoccupied with the stale and the profane, lacking vitality, creativity, and insight, or even outsight. Harassed by unseen circumstances, we remain tethered to existential ghosts that roam our subconscious.

Chaos and distress are so persistent that they become homeostatic, a grim "normal" sustained by unexamined patterns of thought, feeling, and being. These entrenched cycles of relating, behaving, and engaging only serve to reinforce the dissonant reality of our unaware state. Breaking free from this flat circle of existence often requires something jarring, even traumatic, to intervene, a rude awakening that shakes the foundation of our perceived stability.

TRACE emphasizes the importance of cultivating awareness as a means of escaping automatic patterns and living with greater purpose.

In terms of health, awareness is about understanding what your body, mind and spirit genuinely need rather than following blanket rules. Consider someone who becomes mindful of their stress levels and recognizes the impact stress has on their physical and mental health. Awareness allows them to identify patterns, such as reaching for junk food when stressed, and equips them to make healthier choices. It enables them to listen to their body's cues, make informed decisions, and prioritize well-being.

In the pursuit of authentic relationships, awareness deepens our connection to ourselves, others, and the natural world. It nurtures empathy by allowing us to understand another person's perspective, enabling thoughtful responses rather than emotional reactions. Imagine a couple learning to interpret each other's nonverbal cues, using awareness to communicate effectively and prevent misunderstandings.

For many, chaotic and repetitive relational patterns feel inescapable, often going unnoticed or unexamined. Constant exposure to superficial and tumultuous interactions can make these experiences seem normal, masking the possibility of deeper, more meaningful connections. True relational quality is a dialed frequency, one accessible to those willing to delay gratification and transcend the self-indulgent allure of unchecked attachment needs and desires based on fear. Through awareness, we unlock the potential to break free from these cycles and cultivate relationships grounded in depth and authenticity.

In your enterprise, which includes professional and educational pursuits and financial security, awareness enhances decision-making by helping you see not only the immediate effects of your actions but also the long-term implications. For example, you might notice a pattern in the times when you're most productive at work versus the times when you're prone to burnout. Recognizing these rhythms helps you understand why these fluctuations are occurring, manage your workload more effectively, and align your actions with both personal and professional goals.

In regard to recreation and recovery, awareness when applied mindfully allows us to savor the present moment, transforming recreation into a source of rejuvenation and balance. Whether it's a walk in nature, traveling, creating, the laughter of loved ones, or quiet moments of solitude, mindful awareness restores energy, inspiration, and a sense of flow with oneself, others, and the natural world.

If an activity leaves you feeling drained, stuck, or regretful, it may not serve its intended purpose. Use mindful awareness to critically evaluate and refine your approach to recreation and creativity, ensuring it aligns with your goals for recovery, leisure, and personal growth. With mindful awareness, recreation becomes not just a break from routine but a vital pillar of well-being within the HEART framework.

Lastly, awareness is key in pursuing transcendent purpose and meaning, as it requires ongoing self-reflection. Staying aligned with your HEART values and adjusting to shifts in your personal philosophy will help keep you on track. Awareness helps you periodically assess whether your actions reflect the person you strive to be and whether you are making choices that feel meaningful and authentic.

Without awareness, however, one risks drifting into a sense of purposelessness and chaos. This often manifests as feeling stuck or looking back with regret, grieving missed opportunities or the selves we could have been. This grief may stem from mourning the potential once held but now lost due to unforeseen outcomes or choices left unmade.

When we lack clarity and self-awareness, a subconscious state of ennui frequently becomes lodged in our psychological blind spots. Like a splinter buried deep, it eludes conscious retrieval, leaving us in a state of subtle but persistent irritation. Awareness helps uncover these hidden barriers, transforming latent grief into actionable insight and perhaps even redemption.

In TRACE, awareness becomes a compass, helping you navigate each HEART facet with intention. The practice of cultivating awareness reveals a spectrum of choices and responses, opening doors to change that may have previously gone unnoticed. By practicing self-reflection and embracing mindfulness, you gain the clarity needed to create a life of depth, purpose, and alignment.

Control

Control represents agency, the ability to take meaningful action toward your goals while accepting that there are areas where you lack control. In TRACE, control doesn't imply eliminating uncertainty; instead, it means recognizing where you can exert or yield influence and where you need to let go. This adaptive mindset fosters resilience, seamlessly aligning with the principles of HEART.

In the context of health, for example, you can control habits around fitness and diet while accepting certain factors that are outside your control, such as genetic predispositions. By focusing on what you can influence, you strengthen your sense of agency and maintain healthier, more adaptable priorities.

Within the TRACE framework, control refers to our capacity to exert agency and influence over our circumstances, though it's not about controlling every aspect of life but rather about mastering the areas where you can make meaningful impact. Control complements awareness by ensuring that your actions reflect your intentions and remain grounded in your HEART values.

The keyword when it comes to control is *agency*—the ability to act and influence one's circumstances to the outcomes one desires. Agency is not simply about control over external events; it's the internal capacity to make deliberate choices and take ownership of those decisions. For example, a creator navigating a highly competitive market exercises agency by choosing to focus on authentic self-expression, aligning their efforts with personal values rather than succumbing to external pressures.

Control, often associated with determination and purpose, gives us a sense of agency and direction within the HEART framework by anchoring our actions to clearly defined objectives. Determination fuels our persistence, while purpose ensures our efforts align with our core values and the broader goals of the framework. It serves as our North Star, guiding us toward attaining our aspirations.

Now, consider the role of awareness in control. Part of being adept at control is recognizing when things are patently out of our control. This might mean accepting unpredictable market shifts, unforeseen setbacks, or the actions of others beyond our influence. By identifying these situations, we can focus our energy on what remains within our power to change, fostering resilience and clarity in decision-making.

This informed awareness of a lack of control is neither hopelessness nor powerlessness; rather, it represents a different kind of agency—controlling how we choose to perceive the situation at hand. It allows us to stay open to new possibilities while confronting the reality of our current circumstances. Through reflection, we can assess whether our actions align with our values and objectives. This process also uncovers hidden assumptions we may have made based on incomplete or outdated information, helping us recalibrate our decisions.

For example, in the realm of health, control enables you to establish routines and make conscious choices about what you eat, how you move, and how you care for your mental well-being. You're empowered to choose foods and exercises that support your health goals and maintain a consistent routine. This kind of control doesn't restrict but instead creates a sense of stability and direction in your approach to health.

In relationships, control involves setting boundaries that protect your energy and values, ensuring interactions are respectful and mutually fulfilling. It means choosing your mindset, how you behave and how you feel. Moreover, with a clear understanding of your personal needs and values, control in this area allows you to foster connections that contribute positively to your life and reduce exposure to those that drain or diminish you.

In your enterprise pursuits, control is about steering your efforts toward goals that align with the HEART framework. It involves planning and goal setting to navigate challenges effectively and prioritizing tasks that contribute to your long-term objectives. For instance, one can control the outcomes of their financial security by choosing an education that leads to a career and professional relationships that give access to their desired lifestyle.

When it comes to recreation and recovery, control allows you to allocate time for meaningful leisure, choosing activities that genuinely replenish you. This conscious approach to relaxation ensures that you maintain a healthy balance, providing a reprieve from daily stressors and keeping burnout at bay. It means choosing our recreational outlets wisely and ensuring they restore vitality, relaxation, inspiration, and childlike wonder.

Control also plays a pivotal role in fulfilling one's transcendent purpose and meaning. By setting clear goals and breaking down your pursuit of your goals into manageable steps, you can take purposeful action toward your aspirations. Whether it's advancing in a cause or committing to personal growth, a strong sense of control helps you remain aligned with your HEART, stay resilient, and persevere even in the face of setbacks.

In short, control in TRACE emphasizes proactive choice, enabling you to engage with each aspect of your HEART intentionally. By avoiding being reactive and focusing on what you can shape, you cultivate a powerful sense of agency that propels you forward. Control, when balanced with awareness, creates a pathway toward a life rooted in stability, purpose, and resilience.

Evolving

Evolving is the catalyst for growth and transformation. As a component of TRACE, evolving reminds you that transformation, whether of your habits, beliefs, or circumstances, is an ongoing process essential for achieving your goals.

For example, a purpose-driven person may find their values or priorities shifting over time. By embracing this evolving, they stay aligned with their true self while making adjustments that keep them authentic to their vision and principles. When you embrace change, your priorities remain a dynamic reflection of your true aspirations and the evolving paths you take.

Embracing Change: Evolving within HEART

Change, as part of the TRACE framework, signifies growth and transformation. It's the driver of our evolving within each facet of HEART, ensuring that progress is not only possible but sustainable. Embracing change means stepping out of familiar routines and mindsets to welcome new ways of being that align more closely with your values, principles, and ultimate purpose.

The journey toward meaningful change begins with recognizing the dissonance between who you are and who you wish to become. Unfulfilled expectations and incomplete stories about our lives can leave us desperate, reeling from the sense that time is slipping through our fingers like sand through the neck of an hourglass. This longing for change can spark a storm of thoughts and emotions as unrealized goals feel daunting, buried beneath mounting responsibilities and the weight of deferred dreams.

To silence this mental turmoil, take the first step: ground your thoughts through the simple yet profound act of writing. Journaling transforms internal chaos into clarity. Ask yourself, "Where do I need to go? Who must I become to get there?"

Naturally, we are preoccupied with how much time has passed, but today is the future you once anticipated, and it will soon fade into a memory, becoming last week, then last month, then last year. This fleeting present grants you the power to shape your reality. Your intentional choices now determine the experiences your future self will reflect upon. Evolving hinges on your willingness to act in this moment.

Awareness is the cornerstone of this evolution. It begins with recognizing how far you are from realizing your potential and confronting the dissatisfaction in your life. This dissonance often stems from setting maladaptive priorities, a flawed operating system, that our grasp resists releasing. Identify whether your current operating system arises from personal choices or external factors beyond your control. Can you summon the agency to change, or are there more powerful factors preventing this evolution from naturally taking place? These powerful factors could manifest in the form of a genetic condition you are at the mercy of, or a relationship where the power dynamics are imbalanced to your disadvantage. It could appear in the form of one's source of income where you are relegated to being supplicant to an employer for the sake of a paycheck that may as well be in the form of stale bread and silt-settled water.

Perhaps you find yourself in a state of learned helplessness where an accumulation of misfortune has left you feeling incapable of initiating change despite the presence of opportunities to do so. This pattern of inertia may harden into psychological ossification, where listlessness, agitation, and subdued despair become the norm—your homeostasis.

Paradoxically, this comfort zone, though harmful, feels familiar and safe. The hazards of homeostasis evade your defense mechanisms and internal alarms that normally signal danger as they burrow deep in your blind spots and the cavernous recesses of your subconscious.

Make no mistake: stepping beyond your comfort zone is distressing and is often met with fear and resistance. To navigate this journey, we must develop distress tolerance skills that enable us to endure the psychological and physiological discomfort of change. These tools empower us to explore the unknown, a necessary step in pursuing a life worth living.

For instance, in the area of health, change might involve adopting a new lifestyle to support well-being in harmony with physical, mental, or spiritual needs. When approached mindfully, this type of change allows you to transition gradually, adapting your habits to fit your values and health goals. Change becomes a vital component of HEART as it encourages you to let go of outdated practices or mindsets that no longer serve your physical, spiritual, and mental health.

Relationships also benefit from change, as connections deepen, evolve, and sometimes dissolve and fade over time. Embracing change in relationships means understanding that growth often requires shifts in dynamics, communication, and boundaries. You may find that some connections strengthen as you adapt to new circumstances, while others naturally phase out, creating space for relationships that resonate with your present goals and values.

Regarding your enterprise, career growth and personal development hinge on your ability to evolve with changing goals and challenges. When aligned with HEART, change in your professional sphere may include taking on new responsibilities, shifting career paths, or seeking further education. Each step forward, although not without its challenges, builds resilience and enriches your journey, helping you approach your career as a dynamic, purpose-driven facet of your life.

For those seeking recreation, and recovery, change is a return to the childlike joy inspired by play, curiosity, creativity, and connection. Whether through self-reflection, building meaningful relationships, or exploring the world around us, engaging in recreation and recovery can unlock transformative experiences unavailable without such leaps of faith. Within HEART, embracing change means incorporating lightness and adaptability into life through leisure and self-care. This approach ensures that recreation, and recovery remain enriching, dynamic, and fulfilling, aligned with our evolving needs.

In the pursuit of transcendent purpose and meaning, change represents the evolution of one's mission, vision, and story. It requires adopting a new habitus, a way of being that reflects growth, transformation, and authenticity. This intentionality means shaping how we think, feel, act, and interact with the world, grounded in an awareness of our unique position, strengths, and challenges. To thrive, we must actively craft a resilient self that is capable of withstanding the changes that life will bring.

Bringing TRACE to Life

With TRACE—Time, Resistance, Awareness, Control, and Evolving—you now have a structured, adaptable tool that works hand in hand with HEART, bringing clarity, intention, and resilience to your life's journey. Each element of TRACE helps you deepen your self-awareness, understand the obstacles and opportunities around you, and make intentional progress toward meaningful goals. TRACE's purpose is not just to guide you through challenges but to help you continually adapt and grow through life's ever-shifting landscape.

In the next chapter, we'll go deeper, applying each TRACE element to the individual facets of the HEART priorities—Health, Enterprise, Authentic Relationships, Recreation and Recovery, and Transcendent Purpose and Meaning. As we break down how Time, Resistance, Awareness, Control, and Evolving relate to each area, we'll look at real-life scenarios and actionable strategies to integrate these principles into your daily life. This focused approach will empower you to turn your HEART priorities into a living, evolving blueprint for a purposeful, fulfilling, and eudaimonic life.

Pause and Reflect

Some reflection questions to help you on your HEART journey:

- What core values drive your life in the dimensions of Health, Enterprise, Authentic Relationships, Recreation and Recovery, and Transcendent Purpose and Meaning? List them and place the list somewhere visible until you can commit these values to memory.
- How do these values align with your current goals and actions? Can you see yourself adjusting your values as you set your HEART priorities?
- List one strength and one area in need of improvement in each of your TRACE processes. Then, simply reflect on how recognizing these factors can lead to progress in each of your HEART priorities.
- What specific techniques or practices can you implement to deepen your awareness within the dimensions of your HEART priorities?
- How can you realign your small-t time to serve your larger purpose? What small actions can you take each day to ensure that your time is not just spent but invested in the things that truly matter?
- How can you discern between resistance that demands persistence versus resistance that signals misalignment?
- Are you responsible for your own life? If not, who is?

Prescribed Philosophies

- Practice viewing time as an investment rather than an expense. Every moment either compounds toward growth or drifts into entropy.
- True awareness is not just self-reflection but requires detached self-observation without immediate judgment.
- If you look closely, you will see that everything is transcendent. Untether yourself from time—you are witnessing the story of your own life.
- Seek a purpose that aligns with your highest virtues, not just external validation or transient goals.
- Sustainable success is about harmony, not just relentless ambition. Time for work, rest, and play should exist in synergy.
- You are responsible for your responses, interpretations, and actions, regardless of external circumstances.
- Resistance is informative. It is a signal, not a stop sign.

CHAPTER 5

Applying TRACE to HEART

"We delight in the beauty of the butterfly, but rarely admit the changes it has gone through to achieve that beauty."[15]

—MAYA ANGELOU

Now that we've explored the importance of creating a framework and foundational elements of TRACE, it's time to bring these tools into everyday life and begin building a road map that brings alignment, direction, and authentic growth to each facet of your journey.

We'll break down each element of TRACE—Time, Resistance, Awareness, Control, and Evolving—and look at how these principles align with the five facets of HEART: Health, Enterprise, Authentic Relationships, Recreation

---

15 Maya Angelou, Rainbow in the Cloud: The Wisdom and Spirit of Maya Angelou, Random House, 2014, p. 97.

and Recovery, and Transcendent Purpose and Meaning. Each facet will be addressed with real-life applications and strategies to bridge theory and practice, helping you build a stronger framework system aligned with authentic, purposeful living. By the end, you'll have a clearer understanding of how these tools work together to help you pursue your life goals, handle challenges effectively, and make choices that align with your values.

Let's dive into each component of TRACE and see how it works in tandem with HEART.

Understanding the Role of HEART in TRACE

To live with intention and purpose, it's essential to integrate TRACE into the five core areas of HEART. Each TRACE component serves as a guide to navigating life's most meaningful pursuits, offering practical tools for overcoming obstacles, setting goals, and making progress in alignment with your priorities.

To build a life of enduring balance and fulfillment, it's vital to strengthen and lengthen the foundational pillars of your well-being. TRACE provides the road map to support these priorities, guiding you toward sustainable growth, purpose, and holistic vitality.

- **Health:** Strengthen and lengthen your body, mind, and spirit through intentional practices that promote distress tolerance, flexibility, and lasting well-being.

- **Enterprise:** Strengthen and lengthen your professional impact, financial security, and commitment to lifelong learning, ensuring sustained success.

- **Authentic Relationships:** Strengthen and lengthen your connections with yourself, others, and the natural world, fostering genuine, lasting engagement.

- **Recreation and Recovery:** Strengthen and lengthen your capacity for recreation, recovery, and creative expression, ensuring balance and renewal in your life.

- **Transcendent Purpose and Meaning:** Strengthen and lengthen your journey toward self-actualization, purpose, and the guiding narrative of your life.

Applying TRACE to each facet of HEART makes you more resilient and adaptable, empowering you to live with greater clarity and alignment in every area of your life.

Understanding the Role of TRACE in HEART

Now, let's look at how TRACE shapes each of HEART's essential facets.

Time: The Foundation for Setting Goals in Each HEART Priority

Time is the foundation for goal setting across all of HEART's priorities and an invaluable investment. Each area requires a conscious approach to time, an irreplaceable resource that shapes your experience, progress, and personal evolution. Here's how time applies across the five HEART priorities

- **Health and Time:** Effective time management in health isn't just about scheduling workouts or meal plans; it's about dedicating quality, undistracted time to nourish your physical, mental, and spiritual well-being. For example, a consistent fitness routine is truly effective only when you're fully present and engaged. Instead of viewing health routines as checklists, prioritize presence and consistency, which will make your routines more enjoyable and effective.

- **Enterprise and Time:** Time well invested impacts career growth in three ways: it is how you pursue your professional goals, plan for your financial well-being, and make space for ongoing learning. Schedule time regularly to update your skillset, explore courses, or engage in networking that aligns with your career trajectory. This ensures you remain adaptable and competitive while securing a lifestyle that suits your needs.

- **Authentic Relationships and Time:** Relationships flourish when you devote both quality and quantity time to meaningful connections. Instead of squeezing in interactions between other priorities, set aside time for deeper engagement. Regular rituals, such as social gatherings, functions, and check-ins, can form a strong foundation for long-term relationships.

- **Recreation/Recovery and Time:** Recovery requires intentional time allocation for rest and play. Are you truly prioritizing the activities that recharge you? Set aside time for leisure, whether it's reading, traveling, or engaging in creative pursuits. Integrating leisure into your routine will not only refresh you but also fuel your effectiveness in other priorities.

- **Transcendent Purpose and Time:** Purpose requires a significant time commitment, not just scheduled moments, but consistent integration of purposeful actions into your daily life. Revisit your long-term vision each morning or reflect on your actions at night through journaling. By connecting your time with your "why," you align your daily choices with your overarching purpose.

Resistance:
Recognizing and Overcoming Barriers Across Priorities

Resistance, both internal and external, is inevitable and often acts as a roadblock to personal growth in each area of HEART. But what if you could turn resistance into a good outcome? You can, and it starts with self-awareness.

Identifying resistance is the first step in using it to build strength and adapt. Resistance might manifest as self-doubt, procrastination, fear, or external obstacles like societal expectations or time constraints. Here's how resistance shows up in each facet, with tips for addressing it:

- **Health and Resistance:** Resistance can appear as mental blocks or physical inertia, the desire to stay comfortable rather than push forward. Overcome this by defining a few non-negotiable habits, such as daily movement, meal prep, and practicing mindfulness. By committing to healthful routines, you build momentum and discipline that fuels your growth.

- **Enterprise and Resistance:** In your career, resistance can show up as impostor syndrome, fear of failure, or burnout. Combat this by breaking large tasks into manageable steps and focusing on the skills and values you bring to the table. Seek mentorship or professional guidance to help navigate challenges and keep you aligned with your goals.

- **Authentic Relationships and Resistance:** Resistance in relationships may appear as avoidance or communication breakdown. Identify patterns such as poor boundaries, emotional withholding, or reluctance to have difficult conversations. Create dedicated time for open communication, or establish cues with loved ones that signal when it's time for important discussions. By addressing resistance directly, you build stronger, more resilient relationships.

- **Recreation/Recovery and Resistance:** Resistance to recreation often appears as guilt or the belief that relaxation must be "earned." Combat this by scheduling regular downtime without any conditions. Integrate leisure into your life as a necessary investment in well-being, not as an afterthought.

- **Transcendent Purpose and Resistance:** Resistance in purpose may arise from fear or uncertainty, but it's also a sign of growth. Address this by setting small, achievable milestones that align with your values. Revisit your "why" regularly to reignite your motivation, and keep pushing forward even when the path seems daunting.

Awareness:
Cultivating Mindfulness in Each HEART Priority

Awareness is the foundation for growth. Developing a strong sense of mindfulness allows you to respond thoughtfully to life's challenges rather than react impulsively. Here's how awareness applies to each facet:

- **Health and Awareness:** Awareness in health means listening to your body's needs. Practice mindfulness by regularly checking in with your physical, mental, and spiritual states. Are you feeling energized or drained? How do your habits affect your overall well-being? Tune into your body's feedback to make better choices.

- **Enterprise and Awareness:** Awareness in your career means evaluating how your actions align with your professional and financial goals. Are your daily activities truly contributing to your vision? Reflect on how your current choices support your long-term aspirations, and make adjustments when necessary.

- **Authentic Relationships and Awareness:** Awareness in relationships means being attuned to your emotions and those of others. Notice when tension arises, and consider the factors that prompt your responses. This allows you to approach situations with empathy and improve communication, strengthening your relationships.

- **Recreation/Recovery and Awareness:** Awareness in recreation means recognizing which activities genuinely recharge you. Is reading more restorative than watching TV? Are your hobbies fulfilling or draining? Are you able to recognize when the body and mind need to recover in order to prevent burnout? Lean into what brings relaxation, joy, and energy, and make time for these activities in your routine.

- **Transcendent Purpose and Awareness:** Awareness in purpose means regularly connecting with your "why." Journaling or meditating on your values helps you stay grounded in your mission, ensuring that your actions align with your deeper purpose.

Control:
Exercising Agency and Adaptability

Control in your life involves recognizing what you can influence and what you must adapt to. This is true across all the dimensions of HEART. It's about exercising agency while also acknowledging that certain circumstances, especially those outside your direct control, require flexibility and adaptability. Here's how control plays out in each area:

- **Health and Control:** Control over your health involves setting intentional, achievable goals for your physical, mental, and spiritual well-being. This may include taking charge of your nutrition, exercise routine, and mental health practices. It also requires acknowledging when factors such as genetics or environmental stressors are at play. When things don't go according to plan, your adaptability will determine how effectively you can adjust.

- **Enterprise and Control:** Control in your professional life means taking ownership of your career trajectory by making deliberate choices about the skills you develop, the relationships you build, and how you position yourself for long-term success. However, this also involves recognizing that some aspects of your career, such as industry shifts or economic downturns, may be beyond your control. Your adaptability and forward thinking will help you pivot when necessary.

- **Authentic Relationships and Control:** In relationships, control isn't about dominating others but about managing your own responses, setting boundaries, and choosing how you invest your time and energy. Control also means recognizing when a relationship has become unhealthy and having the courage to step back or end it when necessary. This is an act of self-respect and self-love.

- **Recreation/Recovery and Control:** Control in recreation means consciously choosing how you spend your downtime. Are you prioritizing activities that rejuvenate you, or are you allowing yourself to default to mindless distractions? Control also means resisting the temptation to overwork, which can leave no room for necessary recreation and recovery. Giving yourself permission to enjoy rest without guilt is key.

- **Transcendent Purpose and Control:** Control over your transcendent purpose and meaning comes from taking deliberate action in alignment with your core values and long-term goals. This means making conscious choices about where you spend your time, energy, and resources. Although life may throw challenges your way, you have the control to stay focused on your deeper purpose and to continue moving forward despite setbacks.

Evolving:
Growing with Each Step

The final component of TRACE is Evolving. This principle represents the continuous process of growth and transformation. Life is not static, and neither are you. As you work through the other four components of TRACE—Time, Resistance, Awareness, and Control—you will naturally evolve. Here's how Evolving plays out across the five priorities:

- **Health and Evolving:** Your health journey is not a one-time achievement but an ongoing process of self-improvement. As you grow older, your health needs will change, and you will need to adapt your routines to suit your current phase of life. Evolving in health means staying committed to lifelong learning about your body and mind, adjusting as you go, and never stopping your pursuit of wellness.

- **Enterprise and Evolving:** Your career will require continual evolution. Evolving in your career means staying adaptable, continuously improving your skillset, and remaining open to new professional directions that align with your broader life goals. As industries evolve, new opportunities will arise, and you must be ready to evolve with them.

- **Authentic Relationships and Evolving:** Evolving in relationships means understanding that as you grow, so do the people around you. Relationships are dynamic, not static. As you evolve, you may outgrow certain connections or find new, deeper bonds with others. Evolving in relationships also involves being open to change, both in yourself and in others, and learning to grow with mutual respect.

- **Recreation/Recovery and Evolving:** Evolving in recreation means recognizing that your leisure activities will shift as your life changes. What once rejuvenated you might lose its appeal, and you may need to explore new forms of rest, play, and creative expression. Stay open to discovering new ways to recharge and nourish your soul.

- **Transcendent Purpose and Evolving:** Evolving in your transcendent purpose means being open to redefining what fulfillment looks like for you as you continue to engage with the world. Your purpose may evolve as you grow and learn more about yourself and the world. The story you tell about your life will deepen and change as you gain new perspectives.

Integrating TRACE into Daily Life

To truly harness the power of TRACE, it's essential to integrate these principles into your daily routine. Start by making small, intentional changes in each area of HEART. As you do, notice how your sense of clarity, control, and purpose improves. Use each of the TRACE components as a reminder to stay present, stay aligned with your values, and keep evolving toward your highest potential.

Start by setting aside time for deep reflection on each component—Time, Resistance, Awareness, Control, and Evolving—and asking yourself how you're currently applying these principles in your life. From there, identify areas where you can improve or where you need to let go of old habits that no longer serve you.

* * *

TRACE is a powerful tool that helps you navigate your life with purpose and intentionality. By applying it to your HEART priorities, you ensure that each area of your life is aligned with your highest values and deepest aspirations. It's not about perfection; it's about progress and being willing to adapt as you grow. The beauty of TRACE is that it's not a one-time fix but a continuous process, a cycle of growth that helps you evolve into the person you're meant to be.

Remember, life is a journey, and the journey toward becoming your best self is one that requires patience, persistence, and a commitment to continual growth. By integrating TRACE into your daily life, you'll find that the obstacles you face become opportunities for growth, and the goals you set become stepping stones on the path toward your highest purpose and meaning.

With the elements of TRACE now integrated into each area of HEART, you have the building blocks to craft a life aligned with your values, aspirations, and inner truths. In part three, we'll go into detail regarding the importance of each facet of HEART and how you can create a HEART-based system to shed ineffective strategies, behaviors, and ways of thinking and reach your full potential. We will also go into detail about how adopting TRACE processes can facilitate this transformation.

Pause and Reflect

- This week, where did the bulk of your time go: Work? A relationship? Play? Is this healthy?
- Where are you feeling the most friction in your life right now? Is this resistance a barrier to break through or a signal to pivot?
- What unconscious patterns shape your choices? Are they sculpting the life you want, or are you merely tracing over old lines?
- What are you gripping too tightly in an attempt to control? What's the worst that can happen if you let go? Would you survive it?
- In what ways have you already evolved within HEART?
- Which aspects of TRACE can you weave into your day this week—not as an abstract idea but as a lived, embodied practice?
- If your life were in complete harmony with TRACE and HEART, how would it feel? What is the single boldest move you can make today to close the gap between that vision and your present reality?

Prescribed Philosophies

- Every moment spent is either an investment in your fulfillment or a withdrawal from your potential. Choose with intention.
- The discomfort you avoid often holds the lesson you need most. Until you see your patterns clearly, you cannot change them. Cultivate deep awareness to align actions with your values.
- Power lies not in controlling external outcomes but in directing your own energy, focus, and responses.
- Growth requires shedding outdated identities and acquiring and implementing new knowledge.
- The highest fulfillment comes not from chasing meaning externally but from weaving it into your daily life through conscious action and alignment.
- Once you lose control, you're being controlled.
- It's okay to put the load down and rest.

PART TWO:

The Framework

CHAPTER 6

Health Foundations for Mental, Physical, and Spiritual Wellness

"Human infirmity in moderating and checking the emotions I name bondage: for, when a man is a prey to his emotions, he is not his own master, but lies at the mercy of fortune: so much so, that he is often compelled, while seeing that which is better for him, to follow that which is worse."[16]

—BENEDICT DE SPINOZA

I n the pursuit of a life worth living, there is a fundamental cornerstone that cannot be overlooked or underestimated: your health. Physical, mental, and spiritual well-being is the foundation upon which we build our dreams, relationships, careers, and purpose. Without a healthy body

---

16 Benedict de Spinoza, Ethics, Part IV, trans. R.H.M. Elwes (Project Gutenberg, 2013), paragraph 1.

and a sound mind, the path to genuine happiness and fulfillment becomes a long, arduous journey.

This chapter will explore how to use HEART and TRACE to take charge of your health in all dimensions, physical, mental, and spiritual, empowering you to make mindful choices and pursue well-being with purpose. With this guide, you can set meaningful goals for your health and chart a path to a life that truly thrives on well-being.

The Autotelic Personality

As we navigate the complex web of life, our health is a thread interwoven with every aspect of our existence. To create a framework for your health, we first need to embrace the essence of an autotelic personality, an approach that transcends health and resonates throughout the dimensions of HEART and TRACE.

An autotelic personality is characterized by a state of flow in which one is fully absorbed in one's activities, experiencing a sense of timelessness and pure enjoyment in the process itself. Psychologists have discovered that certain traits are commonly found in individuals who tend to experience intrinsic joy in the tasks and challenges they are dedicated to, reaping the rewards of being engaged in the journey itself.

This concept, introduced by psychologist Mihaly Csikszentmihalyi, suggests that we can find fulfillment not just in achieving goals but in the journey toward those goals.

The autotelic personality hinges on characteristics including Clarity, Centeredness, Commitment, Continuous Feedback, Choice, and Challenge. Each trait can be cultivated to aid your pursuit of a life worth living, not just in terms of health, but across all areas encompassed by HEART and TRACE.

- **Clarity** marks the initial step in channeling your autotelic personality. It entails outlining clear and well-defined goals that are genuinely worthy of your pursuit. When it comes to health, clarity is crucial for prioritizing what truly matters. It's about identifying which aspects of your health require attention, then setting specific objectives. You might, for example, aim to achieve a flexible and antifragile mindset, lower your stress levels, or initiate a spiritual practice. Clarity allows you to discern your health-related aspirations so you can design a path to reach them.

- **Centeredness** is the unwavering focus you bring to your health-related endeavors. With countless distractions vying for attention daily, being centered means maintaining absolute focus on the task at hand and minimizing disruptions. This quality is indispensable because it enables you to concentrate on your health goals and filter out the superfluous distractions that don't serve your pursuit. Centeredness ensures that your energy and attention are invested where they matter most, whether in a workout routine, a mindfulness practice, or a balanced diet.

- **Commitment** stands as a testament to your dedication in this journey. An autotelic personality embodies commitment by adhering to a specific mindset and maintaining one's emotional balance and work ethic irrespective of changes in mood, motivation, or obstacles along the way. In the context of health, commitment means embracing the discipline required to stay the course even when initial excitement fades or challenges seem insurmountable. Commitment to your health urges you onward in your pursuit of well-being regardless of the hurdles you may encounter.

- **Continuous Feedback** is your personal system for monitoring and measuring your progress. This component is crucial for self-assessment and growth. By recognizing your advancement in various health-related endeavors, you can objectively evaluate your progress and pinpoint where adjustments are necessary. Continuous feedback helps you remain adaptable and responsive in your approach. When striving for optimal health, it's the ability to track your well-being, whether by assessing your fitness achievements, monitoring stress levels, or observing dietary improvements, that allows you to achieve long-term health.

- **Choice** forms a cornerstone of an autotelic personality. It's the ability to select tasks of value, those that closely align with your purpose, passion, and long-term objectives. In the realm of health, choice means opting for activities you genuinely enjoy and are willing to engage with consistently, despite obstacles. It involves making decisions that contribute to your overall well-being, whether by selecting nutritious foods, incorporating enjoyable exercise routines, or embracing stress-reduction practices.

- **Challenge** means engaging in tasks that provide the right degree of difficulty. Challenging tasks require unwavering focus, which is facilitated by the other Cs—Clarity, Centeredness, Commitment, Continuous Feedback, and Choice. These challenges are neither too easy nor too hard; they are the sweet spot that keeps you engaged. Challenges keep your health journey invigorating and ensure you remain invested in your pursuits.

These characteristics, which are at the core of an autotelic personality, create the groundwork for self-reflection. They empower you to define clear health goals, concentrate your focus, embrace unwavering commitment, stay adaptable through continuous feedback, make valuable choices, and seek the right degree of challenge. We discuss them here to help you internalize these characteristics, but they don't stop at health; they are equally relevant and effective across all dimensions of HEART and TRACE, enhancing your personal development and empowering you to lead a life of purpose and meaning.

Self-Reflect on Your Health

When embarking on self-reflection in the physical dimension of your health, think of it as tending to the temple of your body. Begin by contemplating your current physical well-being with honest introspection. Consider your physical condition, fitness, and overall health.

Ask yourself questions like: *Am I eating a balanced and nutritious diet? Do I engage in regular physical activity that promotes strength and stamina? How well am I managing stress? Am I getting enough sleep?* Take an objective look at your physical habits, as they play a pivotal role in your overall health.

This assessment requires a mindful and intentional relationship with your body. Many of us live our lives without questioning the effects of our environment, family history, relationships, emotions, thoughts, illnesses, accidents, traumas, and overall life experiences on our body, mind, and spirit. This exploration demands a meaningful connection with, and to be blunt, a radical love for, our bodies. Are you comfortable in your own skin, or do you harbor negative body image issues? Has your body experienced any trauma, whether physical or psychological, that has yet to be addressed? This could include illnesses or disabilities that have significantly impacted your identity and quality of life and may, at one point or another, have caused you significant pain and suffering.

The body remembers everything. In his book *The Body Keeps the Score: Brain, Mind, and Body in the Healing of Trauma* (2014), Dutch psychiatrist Bessel van der Kolk presents extensive research on how the body and mind retain and react to the traumas experienced throughout a person's life.

Self-reflection offers an opportunity to explore the thoughts and emotions tied to yourself, engaging in a hermeneutic exercise to decode the living, breathing enigma of the body, along with all the messages and memories it holds, and foster a deeper connection with it.

Revisiting the metaphor of life as a jungle, ask yourself: Would the current state of your health help you survive? Beyond survival, would your health allow you to thrive? Can you move adroitly through unforgiving, treacherous terrain, protecting yourself from nature's relentless assault on the triarchy—the body, mind, and spirit? Are you resilient enough to navigate life's challenges during the day and still gather around the fire with friends at night to share tales under the moonlight?

The strength of this triarchy is not only a general symbol of vitality but also a signal to ourselves, others, and nature itself that, all things considered, we are resilient, adaptive, and capable enough to explore the mysteries of life and all it has to offer.

The mental and emotional aspects of your health are equally tied to your overall well-being. To self-reflect in these areas, take a closer look at your thoughts, emotions, and how you interpret and conceptualize your experiences both inside and outside of yourself.

Consider your emotional well-being: How do you manage stress, anxiety, and sadness? Do you use strategies to manage these stressors, and do those strategies actually help? Often we neglect to examine how our family history affects our mental fitness, and as a result we may unintentionally repeat patterns that reinforce our ingrained habits, leading to a vicious cycle. Self-reflection here allows you to both examine the emotional tools and strategies you already have and identify areas where they may be lacking. By recognizing your strengths and shortcomings, such as emotional patterns, prompts, and triggers, you can develop a deeper understanding of your inner world.

In terms of mental health, consider your cognitive habits and mindset. Do you engage in negative self-talk? Are there recurring thought patterns that hinder your well-being? Self-reflection can help you identify the current mindset, emotions, and behaviors that shape your experience and empower you to transform them into a growth-oriented and adaptive mental framework.

Religion and Spirituality

Religion has been one of the most influential forces in shaping human history, defining entire cultures, influencing political ideologies, and providing frameworks for family, gender roles, and life cycles. Religion has given rise to countless rituals and practices, from birth rites to funeral customs, that serve to guide us through the human experience.

For many, religion provides a bridge to a relationship with the divine and a sense of meaning in an incomprehensibly vast universe. This connection can offer great solace, acting as a key to the mystery of existence.

Those in power, often under the banner of religion, have profoundly shaped our understanding of self, thought, behavior, and our relationships with others and nature. They have packaged these influences as a bridge to the spiritual, a connection to the great unknown within an unfathomable universe. For many, this supplication to the unknown is a balm for the deep, primal fear of consciousness in a vast and enigmatic cosmos. But not for all.

While religion in its many forms has undeniably benefited humanity, its ancient practices often predating modern institutions, its darker consequences cannot be ignored. Unexamined beliefs and dogmatic adherence have eroded individual agency and self-determination. History bears witness to countless wars waged in the name of faith, leading to the loss of innocent lives, the devastation of entire ways of life, and the ruthless exploitation of Earth's resources. The destruction of flora, fauna, and communities with imperious apathy under the guise of piety reverberates through time, shaping the world in ways we experience, often unknowingly, even today.

Curiosity about religion inevitably leads to questions about identity, belief, and purpose. Consider the cognitive dissonance that arises when one begins to doubt doctrines inherited through birth, whether by region, culture, family, or era. How does one grapple with the realization that their religion was chosen for them, a result of circumstances beyond their control? The journey from certainty to doubt demands immense psychological and emotional fortitude. Why would anyone willingly endure the pain of questioning, the risk of ostracism, or the loss of the safety and surety that faith provides? These questions challenge the narratives that define us and reveal how much of our small-r reality rests on unexamined foundations, overshadowed by the staggering capital-R Reality that exists just beyond our perception.

Dear reader, have you ever considered the extent to which religious literature, rituals, symbols, and narratives shape your language, your education, and the governance you live under? Have you critically engaged with your faith, questioning its influence on your perception of both inner and outer reality? If not, could it be that your worldview has been shaped by unexamined assumptions subtly imprinted over a lifetime? Through religion's lens, we often filter emotions, thoughts, and even actions, sometimes passing judgment on others without realizing how deeply these inherited ideals influence us. We must guard against the hubris of unquestioned certainty, the presumption that our beliefs are the sole truth without the scrutiny they demand.

Religion is the structured communal practice of beliefs and customs that connect us to a divine source. *Spirituality*, on the other hand, though sometimes intertwined with religion, is a more personal and often less structured path. Spirituality focuses on finding meaning, cultivating a deep connection to the world, and experiencing an expansive sense of self that transcends the boundaries of ego and identity.

According to Thích Nhất Hạnh, spirituality is not religion but a path to generate happiness, understanding and love while discovering ways to handle life's difficulties where we are.[17]

According to Dr. Maya Spencer of the Royal College of Psychiatrists, spirituality involves the recognition of a sense or belief that there is something greater than oneself, something divine in nature, beyond sensory human experience yet still a part of it.[18]

Researchers Chitra Victor and Judith Treschuk describe spirituality as the pursuit of meaning, quality of experience, and connection to others, nature, community, and a higher power. They add, "Spiritual people love others and connect with others and the higher power or God. Health and well-being are achieved by maintaining a healthy spirit. A healthy spirit is achieved through a healthy lifestyle and connectedness with the higher power or God."[19] With this kind of mindset, it's easy to see how spirituality can play a reparative role in our lives.

Spirituality invites us to deepen our human experience by recognizing the connections that unite us with ourselves, others, nature, and the universe itself. A common theme in spiritual practice is the pursuit of harmony and wholeness. This pursuit is not about achieving perfection but rather about experiencing an integrated self, an alignment of body, mind, and spirit. The values and ethics in spiritual practice support this wholeness, helping us avoid unintentionally maladaptive behaviors that fragment the self and inhibit growth. When we ignore this journey toward wholeness, our health can deteriorate across the physical, mental, and spiritual planes.

---

17   Thich Nhat Hanh, The Art of Living (HarperCollins EPub Edition, 2017), Introduction.

18   Dr. Maya Spencer, "What is spirituality?", Royal College of Psychiatrists, 2012, https://www.rcpsych.ac.uk/members/special-interest-groups/spirituality/publications-archive.

19   Chitra G. Paul Victor and Judith V. Treschuk, "Critical Literature Review on the Definition Clarity of the Concept of Faith, Religion, and Spirituality," Journal of Holistic Nursing, 2019; vol. 38, iss. 1, pp. 107–113.

Reflection on Spiritual Health

Consider how spirituality shows up in your life. Are you aware of your own beliefs, values, and ethical framework, and do they align with how you live your life? Think about the beliefs that feel meaningful to you, whether they are rooted in tradition, intuition, or your own experiences. Reflect on your sense of connection to yourself, others, nature, and the universe, and ask yourself if you feel whole or if certain areas of your spiritual health could be nurtured or strengthened through consistent devotion and practice.

Spiritual health, unlike other areas of well-being, is a lifelong journey that doesn't end or reach a point of perfection. The more you explore and engage with the spiritual dimension of your life, the more you can cultivate a foundation of inner peace, resilience, and self-understanding.

Building a Foundation of Health with HEART

As we've explored in this chapter, your physical, mental, and spiritual health form the essential groundwork for a fulfilling life. By applying the characteristics of an autotelic personality—Clarity, Centeredness, Commitment, Continuous Feedback, Challenge, and Choice—you're developing a mindset that nurtures both resilience and purpose. Through self-reflection, you've started to uncover a deeper connection with your own values, beliefs, and intentions, establishing a clearer understanding of what it means to cultivate genuine well-being.

This foundation is the beginning of a transformative journey. You now have the guiding principles that will help you approach each facet of your health as a means to align with a life worth living. In the next chapter, you'll build on these insights by identifying specific areas of focus and setting meaningful health goals. With HEART and TRACE, you'll be equipped to take practical, empowering steps to achieve and sustain balanced, holistic health.

Pause and Reflect

Some reflection questions to help you on your physical, mental, and spiritual health journey:

- How can Clarity, Centeredness, Commitment, Continuous Feedback, Challenge, and Choice help you design your health priorities?
- How has self-reflection changed your understanding of your physical, mental, and spiritual health?
- Are there any areas of your health that stand out as needing immediate attention?
- How do you practice gratitude and compassion for your body, mind, and spirit?
- List some unhealthy habits you would like to break to promote healing of the body, mind, and spirit.
- How do your current health objectives reflect your core values, and what adjustments might help them align even more closely?
- If I approached my health as a sacred relationship with myself, what would I start doing, or stop doing, today?

CHAPTER 7

Setting Health Goals and Taking Action with TRACE

"Small disciplines repeated with consistency every day lead to great achievements gained slowly over time."[20]

—JOHN C. MAXWELL

I n the last chapter, we explored the foundational aspects of health, reflecting deeply on our physical, mental, and spiritual well-being. With the guidance of the traits of an autotelic mindset, we began uncovering the values and intentions that shape our approach to health.

Now, it's time to put those insights into action. Let's move forward and start shaping your health objectives with intention and purpose.

---

20 John C. Maxwell, The 15 Invaluable Laws of Growth, *John Maxwell's Laws series*, Center Street, 2012.

Set Concrete Health Goals

This next phase will guide you in identifying specific areas for improvement, setting impactful health objectives, and applying TRACE principles to create a sustainable path forward. Here, you'll turn self-reflection into strategy, using HEART and TRACE to structure your health goals with purpose and clarity.

As you move through this chapter, keep in mind that each step is about aligning your health with your values, allowing you to build habits and routines that support a life of lasting health, vitality, strength, and flexibility. Let's dive in and start translating your reflections into meaningful, achievable goals.

Assess Your Current Health Status

Start by taking a comprehensive inventory of your health. This assessment should include your physical, mental/emotional, and spiritual well-being, casting a wide net over the different aspects of your life that contribute to these dimensions.

For instance, in terms of physical health, you might evaluate your exercise routine, nutrition, sleep patterns, and any existing health conditions. When it comes to mental/emotional health, reflect on your stress levels, your emotions, your mindset, and any personal myths—the stories you tell yourself that are based more on assumptions than on truth. And for spiritual health, consider your sense of purpose, your connection to your inner self, and whether your core values align with how you live each day.

Prioritize Areas Needing Attention

After assessing your health, you may notice several areas that could benefit from change. Consider which aspects of your health are causing the most disruption or discomfort in your life. Perhaps your lack of physical fitness is affecting your mental health, or a sense of disconnection is causing emotional distress or even a feeling of emptiness. Prioritize the areas that will have the most impact.

Identify Specific Issues or Concerns

Once you've prioritized, dig deeper into the specific issues that need attention. For example, if mental/emotional health is a priority, you might identify stress and anxiety as recurring issues. Try to understand the root causes behind these challenges: Are there particular situations that amplify your stress? Are certain thought patterns contributing to your anxiety? Identifying these specific challenges can help you direct your energy toward meaningful change.

Connect with Your Values

An essential aspect of identifying areas of potential change is ensuring alignment with your values and life purpose. Consider your values not as abstract beliefs hold but as ethics and priorities expressed through action. Ask yourself how addressing these health issues resonates with your core values, and then engage in actions that reinforce these ideals.

For example, if you value well-being and vitality, identifying and engaging in specific activities that reinforce this belief will keep you motivated to stay on track. And don't be discouraged if you find yourself questioning, "What are my values?" Many of us were introduced to values from outside influences— family, culture, and community. These values may need to be re-evaluated to determine whether they truly resonate with who you are today and who you're trying to be in the near future.

Seek Professional Guidance if Needed

Self-reflection and assessment are essential, but knowing when to seek professional guidance is equally important. If you encounter complex health issues or areas where you lack expertise, consult healthcare professionals or specialists to get tailored support and recommendations. Whether you're managing a chronic health condition, addressing specific mental health concerns, seeking spiritual guidance, or starting a fitness journey, expert advice can offer you clarity and structure as you work toward improved health.

By systematically narrowing down your broad spectrum of health considerations into manageable, specific areas that align with your values and purpose, you set the stage for creating actionable health objectives. These objectives will form an essential part of your HEART plan and will integrate with TRACE metrics. Through this process, you'll be establishing a holistic, purpose-driven approach to improving your health and well-being.

Creating a Framework for Your Health Objective

Now that you've pinpointed specific health areas needing attention, it's time to craft a health-oriented framework objective aligned with the TRACE principles: Time, Resistance, Awareness, Control, and Change. These principles will guide you in setting a clear, impactful, and sustainable health goal.

Impact of Health on Enterprise

Good health is foundational to sustaining the energy, focus, and resilience needed for professional success. Here are several reasons why.

- **Benefits:** Physical health enhances energy levels, while mental and spiritual well-being improve clarity and creativity, allowing for better decision-making and problem-solving.

- **Consequences of Neglect:** Physical illness and mental fatigue reduce productivity and cognitive function, while spiritual disconnection leads to existential uncertainty, impairing long-term professional focus and satisfaction.

- **Opportunity Costs:** Neglecting health leads to chronic stress and burnout, diminishing professional potential and causing missed opportunities for personal growth.

- **Short- vs. Long-term Impact:** In the short term, sacrificing health for work may seem effective, but over time the accumulation of stress, mental strain, and physical decline limits professional performance and fulfillment.

Impact of Health on Authentic Relationships

Physical and mental well-being deeply affect the quality of our relationships, both with others and with ourselves.

- **Benefits:** Good health fosters emotional stability, enabling deeper connections and more empathetic interactions with others. Spiritual health, being aligned with one's sense of purpose, strengthens authenticity in relationships, allowing for genuine, supportive connections.

- **Consequences of Neglect:** Poor health leads to emotional withdrawal, irritability, and detachment from others, while spiritual disconnection causes a sense of emptiness and inauthenticity in relationships.

- **Opportunity Costs:** Failing to care for one's health can lead to emotional exhaustion and isolation, which may strain relationships and ultimately weaken bonds with others and oneself.

- **Short- vs. Long-term Impact:** Short-term neglect might not immediately affect relationships, but over time, the emotional strain caused by declining health and spiritual dissonance erodes trust, intimacy, and connection.

Impact of Health on Recreation and Recovery

Physical and mental health enable meaningful engagement with rest, recreation, and creative pursuits. Spiritual health also plays a key role in finding peace and purpose through restorative activities.

- **Benefits:** A healthy body and mind allow for deeper relaxation and enjoyment of leisure activities, while spiritual health fosters a sense of renewal and fulfillment in recreation.

- **Consequences of Neglect:** Poor health limits participation in fulfilling activities, and spiritual disconnection leads to a sense of aimlessness, making even restorative practices feel empty.

- **Opportunity Costs:** Neglecting recovery reduces creativity and zest for life, stunting personal growth and well-being.

- **Short- vs. Long-term Impact:** While pushing through without recovery may seem productive in the short term, over time it leads to burnout, diminishing one's physical, mental, and spiritual vitality.

Impact of Health on Transcendent Purpose and Meaning

Our health, physical, mental, and spiritual, forms the foundation for pursuing a sense of transcendent purpose.

- **Benefits:** A healthy body and mind sustain the energy and clarity necessary for aligning with a higher purpose. Spiritual well-being offers the wisdom and connection needed to live in alignment with one's deeper life narrative.

- **Consequences of Neglect:** Physical and mental health struggles limit our ability to engage deeply with purpose-driven activities, while spiritual disconnection fosters a sense of meaninglessness and disorientation.

- **Opportunity Costs:** Ignoring health leads to a reduced capacity for self-actualization and personal fulfillment, limiting the pursuit of transcendent goals.

- **Short- vs. Long-term Impact:** While neglecting health may temporarily allow more time for pursuit of other goals, in the long run it hinders one's ability to align with and sustain a deep, fulfilling life narrative.

By following this health framework approach, you create a health-driven objective that aligns with your physical, mental, and spiritual well-being goals. These objectives serve as the foundation of your health improvement plan, empowering you to integrate the TRACE process effectively for sustainable health and wellness.

Now, let's talk about how to attach TRACE metrics to your health priorities, equipping you with tools to approach your health journey with purpose and intention.

Attach Your TRACE Metrics

To ensure your health objective is not just a vague aspiration but a clear and achievable goal, it's vital to attach TRACE metrics to it. The TRACE framework—Time, Resistance, Awareness, Control, and Change—then becomes your navigational tool throughout your health journey, offering structure and clarity at every step. TRACE metrics become your allies, helping you track your progress, make adjustments, and stay motivated as you move toward your health objectives.

Time

Setting a clear timeframe is essential to shaping your health objective into something measurable and actionable. Define a specific start date and a target deadline for your health goal. With a concrete timeframe in place, progress becomes easier to measure, and you gain a sense of urgency and direction. By organizing your health activities with precision, a timeframe becomes more than just a set of calendar checkpoints, it becomes an investment in the quality of life you're building.

Resistance

In the context of health, resistance includes the obstacles or challenges you may face on your journey toward your health objective. Resistance can take many forms: procrastination, self-doubt, distractions, or even fear.

Recognizing these obstacles ahead of time allows you to prepare strategies for overcoming them, building your resilience in the process. For example, if your goal is to improve mental health by practicing stress management, you may encounter resistance from a busy schedule, work-related stressors, or emotional fluctuations. To navigate these, develop a strategy to counter resistance, such as blocking out time specifically for relaxation or having quick stress-relief techniques at the ready. Devising coping strategies for resistance ahead of time allows you to face the inevitable challenges with a sense of readiness, keeping you focused and committed.

Awareness

Self-awareness is integral to your health journey. By using TRACE metrics, you can measure your progress accurately and see your growth over time. For instance, if your goal involves improving physical fitness, incorporate specific metrics such as tracking daily steps, maintaining a food journal, or using a fitness app to monitor your activity. These metrics provide data that allows you to see your achievements clearly and to understand where adjustments might be needed. Journaling can also be a powerful tool for capturing thoughts and moods over time, revealing patterns in your mental and emotional state that you might otherwise overlook. These regular self-checks become a source of motivation, allowing you to appreciate each step you take toward improved health.

Control

Health objectives should distinguish between what you can influence and what lies beyond your control. By focusing on areas of health where you have agency and accepting circumstances outside your influence, you create a sustainable path to growth and resilience. For example, if your goal is to improve mental health, you might decide to accept genetically inherited conditions and shift your emphasis to managing cognitive processes—challenging and reshaping distortions, embracing constructive truths, and fostering empowering beliefs. These are elements firmly within your control.

By aligning your daily choices within this framework, you take ownership of your mindset and philosophies, equipping yourself to navigate challenges with clarity, purpose, and intention. Objectives that align within your sphere of control empower you to make intentional decisions and maintain consistent progress. Recognizing when professional support is needed is a powerful example of exercising this clarity.

Evolving

Incorporating change metrics into your health objective allows you to recognize and celebrate the positive transformations in your life. If your goal is to enhance your mental clarity and emotional balance, track the changes in your stress levels, emotional resilience, and sense of inner peace. These change metrics become touchstones, providing valuable data that highlights even the smallest steps toward your goal. As you move forward, these changes help reinforce your commitment and remind you of the personal growth you're experiencing along the way.

By attaching TRACE metrics to your health objective, you transform a goal into a comprehensive, structured plan that offers measurable and valuable feedback at each stage. This structure will guide you through any resistance, sustain your awareness, and support each step you take toward meaningful change.

Utilizing Resources for Health Monitoring

A health journey becomes easier when supported by visual aids and digital tools, such as smartphone apps. These resources can help you stay mindful of your TRACE metrics, make consistent self-assessments, and maintain steady progress toward your health objectives.

Visual Aids

Visual aids offer a tangible way to monitor your health progress. Charts, graphs, vision boards, and personal journals make health goals easier to understand and track. If your goal involves fitness, for instance, you could chart your improvements in physical strength, stamina, or flexibility over time. Watching your progress visualized in this way can serve as a powerful motivator, helping you see how each step moves you closer to your objective.

Smartphone Apps

In our digital world, smartphone apps offer diverse tools for tracking health. Many apps cater to specific goals, such as physical fitness, stress reduction, or dietary tracking. Here are some examples of how to make the most of these apps:

- **Fitness Apps:** For physical health objectives, fitness apps provide workout routines, track daily steps, monitor heart rate, and offer guided meditations. These features allow you to keep real-time tabs on your fitness and health progress.

- **Mindfulness Apps:** Mindfulness apps are designed to support mental wellness by guiding you through meditation exercises and helping to reduce rumination. These apps can generate daily or weekly reports, allowing you to observe your mental and emotional state over time.

- **Mood- and Stress-Tracking Apps:** These apps provide relaxation exercises and offer tools for monitoring mood shifts and stress levels. Regular check-ins on these apps can help you assess your emotional health and identify areas that may need attention.

- **Goal-Tracking Apps:** For more general health objectives, goal-tracking apps let you set and monitor your progress in areas of your choice, such as weight loss, sleep routines, or exercise frequency. These apps allow you to easily track milestones and keep a clear view of your journey.

- **Health Diary Apps:** Digital diaries enable daily self-reflection, helping you capture thoughts, emotions, and experiences related to your health journey. This practice can deepen self-awareness and offer valuable insights into your progress.

By using visual aids and smartphone apps, you can transform your health objective into a structured and manageable plan. These tools allow for regular self-checks and real-time data collection on your progress, making it easier to stay motivated and on course. Whether you're monitoring fitness goals, tracking diet, managing stress, or keeping a health diary, these resources provide actionable data that help you make informed choices and adapt to changes as you progress.

Other resources for health monitoring include:

- **Professional Intervention:** A health check-up that includes a physical exam, blood work, and a hormone panel can be an excellent starting point, particularly for those who don't have regular visits with their doctor. This approach provides a precise and comprehensive way to measure health outcomes—something that's beyond the reach of self-assessments or what a layperson can do on their own. These tests give valuable insights into your overall health and can help detect any underlying issues early, allowing for more targeted and effective interventions.

- **Analog Journaling:** Journaling can be a profound tool for self-reflection and health tracking. By using pen and paper, you create a physical record of your progress that feels more personal and intentional than a digital log. The act of writing slows your mind, grounding you in the present moment. This tactile process engages your senses, which fosters a deeper connection with your thoughts and emotions and often enhances clarity and insight. Additionally, journaling by hand can serve as a mindful ritual, helping you regulate stress and cultivate a greater sense of well-being as you document your health journey.

When you integrate TRACE metrics into your health objective, you create a comprehensive, holistic plan that not only drives improvement but also equips you with the tools to monitor and manage your goals effectively. Remember, TRACE serves as your compass, helping you stay on course, adapt to challenges, and ultimately achieve your health goals. Having a clear timeframe, strategies to navigate resistance, consistent self-awareness, a focus on control, and an openness to change primes you for success in achieving your health goals.

Mindset and the Autotelic Personality

At the heart of your health journey is a growth-oriented mindset, and this is where the qualities of an autotelic personality—Clarity, Centeredness, Commitment, Continuous Feedback, Challenge, and Choice—become essential. A growth-oriented mindset, characterized by the traits of an autotelic personality, sets the foundation for meaningful progress and guides you through challenges as you work toward your health objectives. This mindset supports not only your commitment to your goals but also a resilient response to the obstacles you may face.

In cultivating this mindset, your *behavior-set* (the context-dependent actions you take), *emotion-set* (the context-dependent way you respond emotionally), and *mindset* (your cognitive approach) become allies in the process of transformation. As you encounter setbacks, the behavior-set you adopt, whether it's perseverance, adaptability, or creating new habits, helps sustain your progress. Similarly, your emotion-set, the emotionally regulated resilience you build to handle challenges without losing hope or direction, keeps you grounded and focused.

Together, these elements reinforce your autotelic mindset, allowing you to see each challenge as an opportunity for growth rather than a setback. This integration of mindset, emotion-set, and behavior-set enables you to not only reach your health objectives but also to deepen your connection to the values, principles, and purpose that fuel your journey. Embracing an autotelic personality equips you with the inner tools necessary for sustainable, authentic progress, helping you navigate each phase of your journey with greater confidence and fulfillment.

*　*　*

Achieving your health-related goals within the framework of HEART isn't just about hitting numbers or milestones, it's about embarking on a transformative journey. This journey deepens your connection with yourself, enriches your relationships with others, and strengthens your bond with the natural world.

It's a process of embracing change and intentionally crafting a life worth living, one centered on vitality and well-being.

By choosing this path, you're not only improving your physical, mental, and spiritual health; you're cultivating a mindset that reframes obstacles as stepping stones for growth. With health as your cornerstone, you are building a future that reflects your deepest values and dreams, a life that thrives in alignment with who you truly are. Let TRACE and HEART guide and ground you as you design a life rich in well-being, intention, and genuine happiness.

Pause and Reflect

Some reflection questions to help you on your health journey:

- Which specific area of your health—physical, mental, or spiritual—feels most compelling to focus on right now? What makes this area stand out for you?
- When setting a health goal, what timeframe feels both challenging and achievable? How can aligning your timeline with your capacity and aspirations keep you motivated?
- What types of resistance or obstacles have you faced in pursuing health goals in the past? How can you leverage TRACE (Time, Resistance, Awareness, Control, Evolving) to prepare for and navigate these challenges more effectively?
- In what ways has the quality of your health positively influenced other aspects of HEART (Enterprise, Authentic Relationships, Recreation and Recovery, Transcendent Purpose and Meaning)?
- Conversely, how has neglecting health affected these areas?
- How do you plan to monitor your health journey and celebrate milestones along the way?
- How will adopting a growth-oriented mindset, behavior-set, and emotion-set influence your health journey moving forward?

CHAPTER 8

A Framework for Your Enterprise

"Your work is going to fill a large part of your life, and the only way to be truly satisfied is to do what you believe is great work. And the only way to do great work is to love what you do."[21]

—STEVE JOBS

M any of us do not fully appreciate the necessity of a holistic enterprise system until we have experienced painful personal setbacks or witnessed others going through significant academic, professional, or financial challenges. It's through repeated encounters with such difficulties that the profound interconnectedness of continuous learning, meaningful professional fulfillment, and financial security and stability

---

21 Steve Jobs, "Steve Jobs' 2005 Stanford Commencement Address," June 12, 2005, posted March 7, 2008, by Stanford University, YouTube, https://www. youtube.com/watch?v=UF8uR6Z6KLc/.

becomes evident. Recognizing and embracing these interconnected dimensions reveals their essential role in achieving a deeply satisfying, resilient, and eudaimonic life.

Continuous learning is the pulse of personal evolution, reflecting the growth mindset, the belief that intelligence and abilities expand through persistent effort and curiosity. Lifelong learners view challenges as invitations to grow, a mindset that promotes adaptability and resilience. Picture a student or professional continually acquiring new skills, enriching their intellectual capacity, and remaining flexible amid life's ever-changing tides. The dedication to academic and intellectual pursuits fuels innovation and creativity, fostering continuous personal and societal transformation. This guided and relentless pursuit of knowledge directly enhances professional fulfillment by equipping individuals with the skills and perspectives necessary to thrive in meaningful work.

Professional fulfillment emerges when your daily work resonates harmoniously with your intrinsic motivations and authentic values. Psychological theories such as Self-Determination Theory emphasize autonomy, competence, and relatedness as fundamental for genuine satisfaction. Imagine the dedicated educator whose passion transforms everyday lessons into vibrant exchanges of wisdom, enriching generations of students. We spend a significant portion of our lives working, so we must make our work count. When you align your work with your values, routine tasks become purposeful actions, infusing your work with emotional vitality and existential depth. This depth of fulfillment subsequently fosters greater financial stability because meaningful, inspired work often leads to higher performance, enhanced opportunities, and sustained professional growth.

Financial stability is the cornerstone of personal freedom, grounding you in clarity and the security to maintain your chosen lifestyle. Psychologically, financial security alleviates stress and frees cognitive and emotional space for higher-level pursuits so you can embody stoic resilience in the face of life's uncertainties. Stable finances are akin to laying down strong roots for a tree, anchoring you firmly so you can extend outward confidently, reaching toward higher-order goals and opportunities such as philanthropy, travel, and creative ventures without anxiety or hesitation.

Yet, it can be overwhelming to navigate these dimensions of enterprise without clear guidance, inspiring role models, structured plans, or a concrete vision. Lack of clarity often breeds confusion and mistakes, leading to cycles of regret and missed opportunities. Uncertainty regarding professional direction may result in lethargy or burnout from uninspired, misaligned work. Financial ambiguity might foster anxiety and perpetual dissatisfaction, robbing life of joy and spontaneity. Without consistent learning and growth, stagnation sets in, leading to sadness and an unfulfilled existence.

The journey toward a richly rewarding lifestyle is inevitably marked by significant challenges: overcoming fears, facing loss aversion, managing procrastination, and adapting to constant change. Psychological grit, as defined by psychologist Angela Duckworth, provides the internal strength required, an enduring combination of passion and perseverance.[22] Establishing clear visions, structured plans, supportive routines, and effective systems transforms intention into reality, reinforcing disciplined progress. Remaining open to serendipitous "luck" aligns philosophically with embracing life's unpredictability, while a strong support network offers guidance, reassurance, and accountability during moments of doubt.

The beauty of successfully navigating these challenges is its profound ripple effect beyond personal gain. Lifelong learners cultivate dynamic environments of curiosity and innovation, benefiting their communities and future generations alike. Professionally fulfilled individuals inspire and guide others toward authentic career paths. Financially stable individuals have the capacity to give generously to charities and philanthropic efforts, positively impacting communities and the broader society.

Thus, enterprise serves as the essential framework for creating the meaningful, flourishing life we envision. It is not merely personal success but collective enrichment, empowering individuals to thrive and, in turn, profoundly enrich the lives around them. While striving for enterprise excellence, it is vital to

---

22 Angela Duckworth, Grit (Scribner, 2016), chapter one.

honor rest and recovery, acknowledging their indispensable role in sustaining long-term fulfillment and effectiveness, a topic explored further in the chapters ahead. Through intentional cultivation of these interconnected dimensions, you build a life that is not just successful but marked by psychological clarity, philosophical depth, and meaningful societal contribution.

The Three Components of Enterprise

Enterprise consists of three core components: professional endeavors, financial independence, and academic pursuits.

- **Professional Endeavors** include your primary career or job, which provides both financial stability and, if one is fortunate, a sense of purpose. It's about finding fulfillment in your work while securing your livelihood, whether it's a calling or simply a means to meet basic needs.
- **Financial Independence** focuses on gaining the freedom to make choices without being limited by finances. This involves achieving milestones like building an emergency fund, setting long term financial goals, or aiming for early retirement. The path includes wisely managing disposable income, creating passive income, and making strategic investments.
- **Academic Pursuits** represent your commitment to ongoing learning, whether through formal education, certifications, workshops, or self-study, to enhance your skills, increase professional value, and improve financial potential.

In essence, your enterprise serves as the professional foundation for future stability, empowering you to live the life you've envisioned and created.

This chapter will guide you in applying HEART and TRACE to your career, moving beyond the conventional idea of simply holding a job. Instead, we'll explore how to cultivate a career that aligns with your values and aspirations, connecting your work to a broader sense of purpose and lifestyle that's both fulfilling and sustainable. Through the HEART approach, you will identify areas for growth, set actionable objectives for professional development, and break those goals down into practical steps to enhance your career satisfaction and personal growth.

Using TRACE as a tool for accountability, you'll ensure that each step you take aligns with your values while enabling you to adapt to challenges along the way. By connecting your professional pursuits to your core identity and aspirations, you will create a path that reflects your authenticity, story, and purpose. This alignment is essential to building a life of meaning, resilience, and balance, one where your career empowers your broader goals and values, rather than limiting them.

Let's begin by taking a closer look at how you can plan your career, uncovering ways to cultivate an enterprise that supports a lifestyle grounded in purpose, clarity, and resilience.

Self-Reflect on Your Enterprise

To plan your enterprise effectively, begin with self-reflection. Consider the quality of life and lifestyle you envision for yourself. How well do your current career choices align with this vision? Those with strong internal motivation and fulfillment in their pursuits are often described as having an autotelic personality, an approach that fosters engagement and satisfaction through the journey itself, not just the destination.

We'll use the principles of an autotelic personality—Clarity, Centeredness, Commitment, Continuous Feedback, Challenge, and Choice—to guide your assessment of your professional life.

- **Clarity:** Examine your career path and current role. Do these choices resonate with your core values and long-term goals? Identifying gaps between where you are and where you want to be is the first step in creating purpose-driven work.

- **Centeredness:** This means being fully present and engaged in your work. Does your daily work allow you to focus on meaningful tasks, or do stress and distractions leave you feeling scattered? Reflect on whether you bring calm and purpose to your responsibilities.

- **Commitment:** Dedication fuels resilience. How committed are you to your career journey, especially during challenges? Consider whether your current path justifies the energy and focus you bring to it.

- **Continuous Feedback:** Regular feedback is essential for growth. Are you receiving input on your performance? Do you clearly understand what's working and what needs improvement? The ability to gauge progress and adjust is key to finding fulfillment in your work.

- **Challenge:** The experience of flow comes when a challenge aligns with your skill level. Tasks that are too simple lead to boredom, while overly difficult ones cause anxiety. The sweet spot is when you're stretched just enough to stay engaged without feeling overwhelmed. Are you appropriately challenged, or is your potential going untapped?

- **Choice:** Reflect on your decisions so far. Are they leading you toward a career that feels meaningful? Do your choices align with your values and help you secure the resources needed for a fulfilling life?

Take time to introspect on how these principles have shaped your career. Reflect on the roles that brought you satisfaction and those that didn't. Consider the moments that stretched you and how they impacted your quality of life. How have your mindset, emotions, and behaviors influenced your approach to work?

Here are some guiding questions to deepen your self-reflection:

- How well does my current career path align with my core values?
- Does my work provide a sense of impact and fulfillment?
- Are there opportunities for skill development and growth in my role?
- Does my income support my lifestyle goals?
- Is my current education level preparing me for future financial and lifestyle needs?
- Is my work–life balance sustainable?

Answering these questions will offer you a clearer view of where you stand and where you want to go. More importantly, this reflection will lay the foundation for your future self, protecting it from the consequences of inadequate preparation.

Identifying Areas for Potential Change

Applying the HEART framework to your career means understanding how your enterprise choices shape the quality of your life and the framework you're building. Your current role and industry impact far more than just your job satisfaction; they influence your mental, emotional, and even physical health. In this section, we'll explore areas within your enterprise that may benefit from change, helping you align your work with your values, goals, and well-being.

Consider these areas as you reflect on where adjustments might enhance your fulfillment and productivity:

- **Lifestyle:** Your enterprise will significantly influence your quality of life, so think about the life you want to live. Does it include a robust employee benefits package? Does it include time to enjoy the fruits of your labor, including fun, meaningful, and joyous times with your friends, family, or even by yourself? Does your profession allow you access to the highest quality of experiences at your disposal? Does your profession provide you with freedom from severe financial stress?

- **Alignment with Values:** Reflect on whether your work supports your personal vision and core values. Misalignment between your career and your beliefs can impact your satisfaction and overall well-being. Are there areas of disconnection, or do you feel your work resonates with what's important to you?

- **Skill Development:** Identify skills or expertise that could enhance your role or open doors to new opportunities. Skill development not only adds value to your career but also increases engagement, making work feel more dynamic and rewarding.

- **Educational Growth:** If your role feels limited, consider whether further education or training could open new pathways aligned with your goals.

Expanding your knowledge base might allow for growth in your current role or offer a route into a different area that better suits your aspirations.

- **Networking:** Professional connections can provide valuable insights, mentorship, and career opportunities. Assess the strength of your current network. Would investing in relationships expand your perspective or reveal new career options?

- **Work Environment:** Evaluate how your work environment impacts your well-being. Do you want to work more or less? Would a remote position, a change in office setting, or even a shift to a different organization improve your engagement and work–life balance?

- **Job Responsibilities:** If your current tasks don't match your strengths or passions, consider ways to reshape your responsibilities. Explore options within your role or even in a different role within your industry that could better utilize your skills and bring greater satisfaction.

- **Entrepreneurship:** For those seeking autonomy, entrepreneurship or freelance work can be a rewarding avenue. Reflect on whether starting your own business or taking on freelance roles would allow you to bring your strengths and passions to the forefront.

This assessment can reveal areas where small or significant shifts might bring greater satisfaction and alignment with your framework. Embracing change doesn't necessarily mean a complete career overhaul. Sometimes, subtle adjustments such as adopting a growth-oriented mindset, pursuing additional training, or shifting responsibilities can make a meaningful difference.

Consider what might improve if you took action to align your role, environment, or skillset with your values. Whether it's a gradual shift in responsibilities, a new educational pursuit, or even a move into a different field, identifying these areas for potential change is a key step toward a purposeful, fulfilling career.

Creating a Framework for Your Enterprise Objective

Now that you have a clearer understanding of the shifts you'd like to make, it's time to apply the HEART and TRACE principles to create a specific enterprise objective. This HEART objective will serve as a blueprint, helping you align your career goals with your values, aspirations, and a purpose-driven path.

Impact of Enterprise on Health

A well-balanced approach to professional, financial, and academic endeavors is crucial for maintaining health. Overwork, neglecting intellectual growth, or compromising on financial stability can harm both physical and mental well-being.

- **Benefits:** Financial stability ensures access to healthcare and wellness resources. Academic pursuits stimulate cognitive health, while professional success supports overall well-being by reducing stress and providing security.

- **Consequences of Neglect:** Chronic stress from overwork or financial strain, along with neglecting intellectual engagement, leads to poor health outcomes, including burnout, anxiety, sleep issues, and physical ailments.

- **Opportunity Costs:** Focusing solely on career or finances at the expense of health and intellectual growth leads to long-term health issues and missed personal development opportunities.

- **Short- vs. Long-term Impact:** While short-term financial rewards or career achievements may feel rewarding, the long-term costs to health and intellectual well-being can be severe and often irreversible.

Impact of Enterprise on Authentic Relationships

Professional and financial stability can enhance relationships, but neglecting academic or personal connections can lead to emotional disconnection and isolation.

- **Benefits:** Financial security enables shared experiences, while intellectual growth fosters deeper, more meaningful connections. A thriving career can also promote positive relationships through professional networks and mutual growth.

- **Consequences of Neglect:** Overwork and financial stress often lead to relational neglect, emotional distancing, and isolation, damaging both personal and professional relationships.

- **Opportunity Costs:** Focusing exclusively on career or finances limits opportunities for meaningful connections and mutual support, undermining both personal growth and relationship quality.

- **Short- vs. Long-term Impact:** In the short term, career success or financial gain may offer satisfaction, but without intellectual engagement and strong relationships, fulfillment will be fleeting. Over time, this imbalance leads to dissatisfaction and isolation.

Impact of Enterprise on Recreation and Recovery

Achieving work–life balance is essential for overall well-being. Neglecting intellectual, professional, or financial health can undermine opportunities for meaningful recreation and recovery.

- **Benefits:** Engaging in academic pursuits enhances creativity and mental recovery. Financial and professional success allows for leisure and travel, contributing to physical and emotional rejuvenation.

- **Consequences of Neglect:** Neglecting professional or academic growth reduces opportunities for rest and relaxation, leading to burnout and diminished life satisfaction.

- **Opportunity Costs:** Focusing solely on work or financial success limits time for intellectual growth and recovery, curbing creativity and long-term well-being.

- **Short- vs. Long-term Impact:** In the short term, working longer hours or prioritizing financial goals may seem productive, but over time, the lack of balance leads to exhaustion, reducing overall satisfaction and productivity.

Impact of Enterprise on Transcendent Purpose and Meaning

When professional, financial, and academic endeavors align with personal values, life takes on greater meaning and makes for an exciting life story.

- **Benefits:** Academic engagement nurtures intellectual fulfillment and influences professional work, which provides opportunities for contribution. Financial stability ensures security, enhancing one's options for creating a life that feels rich in purpose.

- **Consequences of Neglect:** Misalignment between career, finances, academic pursuits, and personal values can lead to dissatisfaction, burnout, time wasted, and existential emptiness.

- **Opportunity Costs:** Prioritizing financial gain or career success over personal values and intellectual development diminishes life's meaning and the opportunity for personal fulfillment.

- **Short- vs. Long-term Impact:** Short-term career or financial achievements may bring stability, but neglecting purpose and intellectual engagement ultimately leads to emotional exhaustion and regret.

Defining enterprise objectives in this structured way gives you practical steps with which to integrate your values and your aspirations, preparing you for a transition that aligns with your vision for a fulfilling career. With the HEART system as your guide, this objective becomes a powerful catalyst that propels you toward an enterprise that reflects your goals and enriches your life.

Attach Your TRACE Metrics

Now that you've defined your enterprise priorities and objectives, it's time to apply TRACE metrics to create specific enterprise objectives with structured milestones so you can track your progress. These metrics will help you stay focused and aligned with your ultimate goal, ensuring that each step you take in your career transition is intentional and purposeful.

Time

Establish both short- and long-term milestones. For example, set aside time each month to review your one-year, three-year, and five-year plans. Break these larger goals into manageable segments to build momentum while balancing your current responsibilities. Revisit and assess your progress at least once a month. Ask yourself if you're investing the time needed to become proficient in your chosen field in order to attain your desired lifestyle.

Resistance

Use a journal to track moments of resistance, whether they are caused by procrastination, doubt, excuses, or external obstacles. Be honest with yourself. Rate each instance of resistance on a scale from 1 to 10, with 1 being the mildest resistance and 10 being the most intense. This will help you identify your biggest challenges and adjust your approach. Also, note instances where you've overcome resistance—these are moments of adaptive resistance. By recognizing your resistance points, you can refine strategies, seek support, or adjust routines to overcome challenges more effectively.

Awareness

Make staying informed a priority. Set weekly notifications for industry news, attend webinars, and connect with professionals in your field. Track your activities, such as the number of connections made, webinars attended, or new resources gathered. Learn as much as you can about your education and career paths. Network with people who have achieved the lifestyle, education, profession, or financial status you desire, and gather insights to guide your preparation. Consider experiences like test-driving your dream car or visiting a potential dream home to elevate your vision to the next level, turning dreams into a tangible reality. Awareness enhances your adaptability, helping you stay attuned to opportunities and trends that support your transition.

Control

Let go of what's outside your control, and focus on controlling what is within your power. This frees up mental and emotional bandwidth to focus on the important things. Regularly evaluate and refine your skills to increase self-confidence and optimize professional viability. Periodically check in on your progress with your priorities, including skills development, professional responsibilities, and financial stability. Use a calendar to keep your schedule organized and ensure a healthy work–life balance.

Evolving

Track your proactive efforts toward securing opportunities. Are you applying for roles, engaging in online work communities, or seeking feedback to improve your approach? Measure these efforts weekly, and be flexible in adjusting your strategy as needed. Tracking your progress allows you to see tangible results, which will build your confidence and sense of momentum toward your goals. If you're in the learning phase, consider joining a study group or working with others more proficient than you. As the saying goes, "Insanity is doing the same thing over and over again and expecting different results." For real transformation to occur, we need to adjust what we do, how we feel, or how we perceive situations.

By integrating TRACE metrics with your HEART objective, you create a system of clear, actionable steps that drive consistent progress. The combination of HEART and TRACE ensures you remain accountable and adaptable, bringing you closer to a fulfilling and purposeful professional life.

Your Enterprise and Your Quality of Life

As you reflect on your journey through the three areas of enterprise (professional endeavors, financial independence, and academic pursuits), it's evident that your choices in academia, career, and financial management profoundly influence your overall well-being and your vision for a fulfilling life. By integrating your enterprise with the principles of HEART and TRACE, you create an approach to work that not only provides financial independence but also fosters a deeper sense of freedom, purpose, and vitality. This structured framework allows you to transform work from a mundane, quotidian task performed in a state of autopilot to a vibrant and meaningful extension of your authentic self.

* * *

Throughout this chapter, you've explored how mindset, emotions, and behaviors influence your work experience. By recognizing these patterns, you gain the tools to make conscious changes that can elevate your professional path and enhance the overall quality of your life. With TRACE metrics in place, you are creating a career strategy that's not separate from the rest of your life; rather, it is integrated within a broader framework, aligning your professional goals with a commitment to holistic well-being.

As you look ahead, embrace the idea that your career is a journey, not a fixed destination. Life's inevitable twists and turns will prompt you to adapt, explore, and redefine what fulfillment means to you over time. HEART and TRACE offer the support you need to navigate these changes, equipping you with a toolkit for flexibility, ingenuity, perseverance, and adaptability.

Pause and Reflect

Some reflection questions to help you on your Enterprise journey:

- What makes your current job fulfilling or unfulfilling?
- How do your thoughts and emotions about work impact your well-being?
- Have you ever received mentorship regarding education, career, or financial independence?

  » If you haven't received mentorship, consider how this might have impacted you, either positively or negatively.
  » If you have, how did the mentorship help or hinder your growth?

- Beyond money or titles, what nontraditional measures of success are most important to you and your community? How do these metrics align with your values?
- Reflect on your fears around education, professional work, and financial status.
- Write down your thoughts, emotions, and behaviors around these fears.

  » Have any of your fears come true?
  » If not, imagine what it would be like if they did. Sit with the thoughts and emotions that arise.
  » If these fears are justified, what can you do now to prevent or reverse these outcomes in the future?

- Periodically fantasize about your ideal education, profession, and financial status. Let your imagination run free, and jot down your dreams without holding back.

  » Have any of these dreams started to come true?
  » If not, would your current self be able to make them a reality?
  » What steps do you need to take now to ensure these dreams become a reality in the future?

CHAPTER 9

Prioritizing Authentic Relationships

"Life is partly what we make it, and partly what it is made by the friends we choose."[23]

—TEHYI HSIEH

In chapter seven, we explored how the HEART and TRACE systems can enhance our health, applying the autotelic characteristics to generate the experience of flow—clarity, centeredness, commitment, continuous feedback, challenge, and choice. But these principles aren't exclusive to health alone; they have the potential to transform all the facets of your life, including relationships.

---

23 Tehyi Hsieh, Chinese Epigrams Inside Out and Proverbs, Exposition Press, 1948.

Our connections with ourselves, others, and even with nature profoundly influence our happiness, well-being, and overall experience. Just as with our health, we can apply the other priorities along with TRACE to elevate and deepen these connections. By reflecting on our relationships, identifying areas that may need adjustment, and setting clear goals, we can strengthen these bonds and better understand our growth within them.

So, let's dive into the world of relationships and discover how its intersection with the TRACE process can help us cultivate connections that bring meaning and positivity to our lives.

Who Are You?

Identity is a mosaic, shaped by countless factors including culture, ancestry, relationships, and the environment. When faced with the question *Who am I?*, many people find themselves grappling with a whirlwind of external influences that clash with their internal values. In a world that constantly tells us who to be, carving out an authentic sense of self can feel like an uphill battle. But identity isn't static—it's a dynamic process shaped by the intersection of biological, psychological, and social forces.

The real issue with *Who am I?* is that it's the wrong question. Identity isn't fixed; it's a shifting, evolving story. A better question might be: *How many "I"s can I be?* This reframing captures the fluid, ever-changing nature of who we are as we adapt to life's shifting contexts and demands. To make sense of this complexity, we can use a simple framework: the *Self within Self*, the *Self within Others*, and the *Self within Nature*. Each dimension offers a lens through which we can better understand the forces that shape us.

The Self within Self

This dimension reflects the relationship we have with our physical body and subconscious mind. Our body's strength or frailty and its flexibility or rigidity directly influence how we experience ourselves and how others experience us. But identity goes deeper than the physical. Unconscious drives often shape how we see ourselves, operating beneath the surface until we actively bring them into awareness. Developing emotional and cognitive intelligence allows us to uncover hidden aspects of ourselves, deconstruct false beliefs, and confront unexamined urges. By doing this inner work, we uncover layers of truth about our body, mind, and spirit that are often obscured by habit or fear.

The Self within Others

No one exists in isolation. Identity emerges and evolves through interactions and feedback from relationships. Parents, friends, siblings, and communities all leave their marks on who we become. Their rituals, boundaries, myths, and even their unspoken traumas seep into our sense of self. Sometimes, these relational forces strengthen us, fostering the development of traits that help us adapt and grow. Other times, relational forces undermine us, leaving scars that shape how we see the world and ourselves within it. By examining the imprints our relationships have left on us, we can decide which relationships to keep, which to heal, and which no longer serve the person we're becoming.

The Self within Nature

Our connection with the natural world reveals itself through the quality of the air we breathe, the region or environments we inhabit, the water we drink, and the food we eat (including the flora and fauna we interact with and consume). All these things play roles in shaping who we are. But beyond these tangible elements, there's something profoundly grounding about being in nature. Research in the field of ecopsychology shows that time spent in natural environments can restore mental clarity, foster resilience, and deepen our sense of meaning. When we're disconnected from nature, we risk losing that harmony, which in turn erodes both our well-being and our sense of self. Reconnecting with nature isn't just restorative; it's a way of revealing and remembering a part of ourselves that often gets lost in the noise.

The Self within Self, the Self within Others, and the Self within Nature remind us that who we are isn't static, but fluid—a reflection of our internal processes, our relationships, and our environment. By understanding these dimensions and the feedback exchanged through our interactions, we can begin to untangle the web of influences that shape us and move closer to the person we're meant to be. Remember, the question isn't *Who am I?* but rather *Who am I becoming?*

Self-Reflect on Your Relationships

Our mindset, behavior, and emotional responses all profoundly influence how we perceive and engage with others. Beliefs about ourselves and others, past experiences, and current emotional states shape these interactions and can either enrich or complicate the quality of our relationships.

When you approach relationships with a positive mindset, you're more likely to act with openness and goodwill. Conversely, carrying negative beliefs or unresolved emotional baggage can create barriers that hinder healthy, meaningful connections.

Reflecting on our relationships means thinking about how we act, react, and interact with ourselves and others, including:

- Family members
- Friends and acquaintances
- Romantic partners
- Colleagues
- Mentors and role models
- Teachers
- Community members

When you begin to self-reflect, start by examining your general approach to relationships.

- **Explore Self-Image and Perception:** Think about how your self-image might affect your interactions. Do you feel confident, assured, and ready to connect with others, or do doubts and insecurities impact your relationships?

- **Examine Your Attitudes:** Reflect on your attitudes toward those around you. Do you naturally approach others with trust and openness, or do caution and judgments based on past experiences affect your connections?

- **Recognize Patterns:** Patterns in behavior, thoughts, and emotions often shape our interactions with others. Do you understand your temperament and personality styles? Are you generally calm and empathetic, or do you find yourself reacting with heightened emotion or with fear in certain relational contexts? Do you tend to view yourself and others more positively or negatively? Are you generally trusting or skeptical? Open or guarded?

- **Assess the Influence of Past Experiences:** Reflect on past relationships that might be influencing your current connections. Are there unresolved issues, traumas, or emotional wounds that impact how you attach to others? Research, like the attachment studies led by Mary Ainsworth, reveals how early parent-child interactions can have a lasting influence on attachment styles in adulthood. Where do you fall in the attachment spectrum? Are you securely attached, anxious, avoidant, or fearful-avoidant?

Understanding your own beliefs, attitudes, and relational patterns is a key first step in self-reflection. By gaining clarity on these internal aspects, you begin to consciously enhance the quality of your connections. Next, we'll explore how to use HEART and TRACE to build upon your reflections, fostering positive changes in relationships.

Identify Areas of Potential Change

To assess your relationships effectively, it's essential to start by exploring your perceptions, behaviors, and underlying mindset. Self-reflection and introspection can reveal areas within your relationships that are ripe for change and growth. Here are a few areas to consider as you move forward:

- **Assess Your Roles:** The relationships you form often reflect the different roles or selves you assume throughout your life. Roles like friend, child, partner, parent, colleague, and more naturally come and go as life happens. However, by understanding these roles, you can recognize how specific dynamics impact your interactions with others. For instance, while you may be a fully mature adult, you might still find yourself reverting to a younger version of yourself around family members. This regression could be spilling over into other contexts beyond just one's family. Recognizing these roles enables you to see where relationships may benefit from further development.

- **Recognize Your Personal Worldview:** It's valuable to remember that your view of yourself and others is shaped by various internalized beliefs. Reflecting on how you see yourself—past, present, and future—helps clarify how certain perceptions influence your relationships. What are your core beliefs about the world? Do you feel that others "owe" you understanding, or do you approach relationships with self-sufficiency? A clear-eyed assessment of these beliefs can be transformative, helping you uncover biases, defense mechanisms, and limiting beliefs.

- **Focus on Your Intentions. Be Present:** Intentionality is about engaging in relationships with purpose. It means aligning your thoughts and actions with your personal values and relational goals. Self-reflection helps you clarify this intentionality, encouraging deliberate and healthier connections. Be present. Many of us know the feeling of being distracted, dissociated, or numb when surrounded by others, in nature and even alone by ourselves. Being present takes effort. It's a conscious choice to engage with life fully, resisting the distractions that pull us away from meaningful connection. While there may be comfort in the passivity of sitting in the backseat of our lives, it's vital to understand that when we relinquish our role in steering our relationships, we risk becoming lost in the chaos of unexamined interactions. The true power lies in choosing to be intentional in how we engage with the world, bringing clarity and meaning to every connection.

- **Reflect on Mindset, Emotion-Set, and Behavior-Set:** These factors shape how you relate to others. A rigid approach to relationships can lead to stagnation and resistance, while flexibility fosters empathy and adaptability. Consider where you fall on this spectrum and how it might be affecting your relationships. When you approach relationships with a flexible mindset, you can more easily adjust to changing dynamics and respond to others with empathy.

Self-reflection is the foundation of effective change within relationships. By delving into the various roles you play, examining your worldview, embracing intentionality, and evaluating your mindset, you can start to reshape how you connect with others. With greater awareness, you lay the groundwork for a more fulfilling relational framework.

How Authentic Relationships Affect the Other Elements of HEART— Creating a Framework for Your Authentic Relationships Objective

With these insights in hand, it's time to translate self-awareness into actionable goals by creating a framework for your relationships. This objective helps clarify the type of connections you want to nurture with others, with nature, and even with yourself so you can align your goals with your values for personal growth and the well-being of those around you. Here's how each dimension of HEART can help you define and support your relationship priorities:

Impact of Authentic Relationships on Health

Social connections provide emotional and physical health benefits.

- **Benefits:** Strong positive relationships reduce stress, enhance immune function, and improve emotional well-being.

- **Consequences of Neglect:** Social isolation increases anxiety, depression, and physical health risks, including higher blood pressure and weakened immune response.

- **Opportunity Costs:** Without meaningful relationships, individuals face greater emotional strain and health deterioration.

- **Short- vs. Long-term Impact:** While independence may seem appealing, prolonged isolation negatively impacts physical and emotional health.

Impact of Authentic Relationships on Enterprise

Healthy relationships at work/business support professional growth through collaboration and mentorship.

- **Benefits:** Trust and cooperation in work relationships contribute to career opportunities and personal development.

- **Consequences of Neglect:** Poor relational health leads to missed opportunities, workplace conflict, and stagnation.

- **Opportunity Costs:** Focusing solely on work at the expense of relationships limits networking, collaboration, and innovation.

- **Short- vs. Long-term Impact:** In the short-term, focusing only on career might seem effective, but over time it limits professional growth and fulfillment.

Impact of Authentic Relationships on Recreation and Recovery

Shared experiences make recreation more meaningful and fulfilling.

- **Benefits:** Connection with self, others, and nature through activities such as camping, hiking, or surfing enhances relaxation and emotional restoration, making leisure activities more enjoyable.

- **Consequences of Neglect:** Isolation diminishes the emotional benefits of recreation, leaving individuals feeling drained and disconnected.

- **Opportunity Costs:** Failing to integrate relationships into leisure diminishes emotional support and long-term well-being.

- **Short- vs. Long-term Impact:** Solo activities may provide temporary pleasure, but over time, emotional depletion arises from a lack of social connection.

Impact of Authentic Relationships on Transcendent Purpose and Meaning

Meaningful relationships offer support and shared purpose, enriching life's meaning.

- **Benefits:** Relationships deepen the sense of purpose by offering mutual growth, guidance, and shared goals.

- **Consequences of Neglect:** Without meaningful connections, life feels empty, devoid of shared purpose, and often directionless.

- **Opportunity Costs:** Focusing on individual success without fostering relationships hinders personal growth and self-actualization.

- **Short- vs. Long-term Impact:** While personal achievement may seem fulfilling at first, long-term isolation weakens one's sense of connection and belonging.

Attach Your TRACE Metrics

With clear relationship priorities in place, the next step is to look at relationships through the lens of TRACE metrics. Each TRACE component will highlight potential relationship goals and ways to track your progress toward them. This makes your goals structured, intentional, and achievable.

Time

In the TRACE process's Time dimension, prioritize quality time with the people and activities that matter most. Since time is finite, be strategic. Attach measurable metrics to your system, for example, commit to spending uninterrupted hours weekly with a partner, friend, or family member to foster meaningful connections through shared activities or conversations, and track your progress by journaling about the experience.

Equally important, reclaim time by setting boundaries against draining or aimless interactions. Ask yourself: *How do I want to experience my time, whether alone or with others?* Use this reflection to align your choices with your values and goals.

Finally, balance these commitments with alone time to nurture self-reflection and growth. A strong relationship with yourself is essential for cultivating thriving connections with others.

Resistance

Resistance in relationships often manifests as unresolved tension, misunderstandings, or a lack of effective communication skills. For most of us, the sources of resistance are not immediately obvious. They frequently elude our understanding while remaining tangible enough to cause significant problems in our relationships.

To address this, it is essential to:

- Deconstruct thoughts, behaviors, and emotions indicative of internal resistance.
- Develop conflict resolution strategies.
- Practice understanding others' perspectives.
- Cultivate the ability to tolerate distress when circumstances do not align with our expectations or assumptions.
- Adopt a mindset to resolve issues rather than avoid them.
- Focus on open and empathetic communication with others.
- Conversely, actively resist relationships with those who are damaging to or dismissive of your principles and values.

Internal Resistance: A Relationship with Self

While external resistance often impacts how we interact with others, internal resistance plays an equally significant role in shaping these interactions.

Your self-awareness practices should include regular self-check-ins to uncover internal resistances that arise in daily life. This introspective relationship reveals defense mechanisms and fears that shape how we relate to others and ourselves.

Strategies to Explore Internal Resistance

- **Journaling:** Record moments of resistance. For instance, if your goal is to improve assertiveness, identify times you felt anxious about saying no or making a request, and note how this specific pattern has affected the course of your life.

- **Cost-Benefit Analysis:** Examine the pros and cons of speaking up versus remaining silent. Reflect on how each choice impacts your progress toward personal growth.

- **Measure Growth:** Track progress in overcoming resistance by identifying patterns, celebrating small victories, and maintaining empathy and openness.

Adopting this approach allows you to better understand and address resistance, fostering both relational and personal growth.

Awareness

Increasing awareness in relationships means honing both your self-awareness and outsight. *Outsight* refers to the ability to perceive external things clearly, including understanding others' perspectives, emotions, and behaviors, seeing things from their point of view. This involves not just observation but deep comprehension of the experiences and feelings of others without projection or bias. To deepen this, identify your biases and blind spots. Self-reflection alone isn't enough; seek external feedback to challenge ingrained assumptions and gain a fuller understanding.

One useful exercise is to document how distractions hijack your focus. Track what competes for your attention throughout the day and how often it pulls you away from meaningful engagement. This exercise reveals patterns that hinder your awareness.

Another good goal is to actively listen and remain present when others share their experiences, striving to understand their desires and motivations, both visible and hidden. Relationships evolve, so avoid the trap of expecting full comprehension immediately. The aim is gradual, deeper understanding over time.

To measure progress, engage in a metacognitive exercise. Pay attention to the fluctuations in your own and others' thoughts, emotions, and behaviors. Use journaling or reflection tools to track these patterns. This practice strengthens attunement to your relationships and helps you uncover insights that might have gone unnoticed.

Lastly, cultivate a consistent awareness of the grandeur of the natural world and note how this influences your thoughts, emotions, and overall experience of yourself and others. By immersing yourself in nature, you can enhance your connection to the present moment and gain valuable insights into your internal state. Additionally, explore literature on human behavior to uncover blind spots and expand your self-awareness. Remember, developing deep awareness is an ongoing process, it takes time, patience, and consistent effort to truly grow.

Control

Control in authentic relationships centers on self-regulation, not on manipulating, dominating, or dictating others' actions. It involves managing your reactions, setting clear boundaries, and ensuring your values guide your interactions. Equally important is recognizing when to relinquish control, accepting that some outcomes are beyond your influence.

A practical goal could be learning to say no when necessary or prioritizing self-care by communicating boundaries effectively. Control also involves recognizing when a relationship no longer aligns with your values or vision and taking steps to distance yourself from it, letting go of the need to pursue a fantasy outcome.

To measure your growth in Control, define specific behaviors that honor your values and enhance self-regulation. For example, you might commit to practicing intentional responses during stressful situations, pausing before reacting to ensure your actions align with your values. Regularly evaluate whether your relationships respect the boundaries you've established and contribute to your overarching goals within your HEART priorities.

Evolving

The HEART framework thrives when we commit to personal changes that promote meaningful, healthy, and authentic relationships. These goals can include enhancing empathy, reshaping ingrained beliefs about relationships, setting limits, and adapting to both expected and unexpected outcomes. Tailor each goal to align with your values, fostering both personal and relational growth.

To track your progress, consider using a change metric to help monitor your adaptability in relationships. For example, you could set a goal to engage in one shared activity with a significant person each month. This could be anything from trying a new hobby together to supporting each other's personal development. By actively monitoring adaptability, you can assess how well you navigate changes, track your progress, and adjust your approach to maintain healthy, growing connections.

Building on these goals to evolve in relationships requires flexibility and an openness to dynamic changes. Your objective could focus on cultivating antifragility, emotional intelligence, and a growth-oriented mindset in both individual and relational contexts. Recognize when relationships grow, stagnate, or regress, and make adjustments accordingly. Changes in relationships can be challenging, unearthing both fears and newfound courage.

Our reactions to transitions are shaped by our beliefs about companionship and independence. Embrace changes, allowing yourself to celebrate or grieve as appropriate.

By attaching TRACE metrics to your relationship objectives, you transform aspirations into tangible actions. These metrics provide a structured framework, helping you track, assess, and refine your approach as you cultivate healthier and more fulfilling relationships.

Utilizing Resources for Relationship Metrics

When it comes to tracking your TRACE metrics in relationships, leveraging external resources can provide both structure and support. Resources like counseling, classes, and technology can assist you in maintaining and measuring your progress, helping you build lasting, meaningful connections.

- **Journaling:** Incorporating journaling into relationship-building efforts enhances self-awareness, emotional intelligence, and intentionality, leading to healthier, more meaningful connections.

- **Counseling or Therapy:** Professional counseling offers a structured environment where you can explore time management, address resistance, and build awareness within your relationships. A counselor or therapist can guide you in creating personalized TRACE metrics, providing insights that align with your values and help you overcome specific relationship challenges. In therapy sessions, you'll have a space to reflect deeply, monitor progress, and receive professional feedback on your relational growth. Counseling offers valuable support in understanding your patterns, gaining awareness, and making meaningful adjustments in your relationships.

- **Classes and Workshops:** There are countless workshops, online courses, and community classes focused on relationship building and self-awareness. These can offer practical skills and tools for measuring and managing TRACE metrics. Many workshops encourage participants to practice emotional awareness, build healthy boundaries, and enhance communication, creating opportunities for hands-on learning. Additionally, such classes can facilitate group discussions and practical exercises, helping you apply TRACE principles to real-life situations while benefiting from shared experiences with others.

- **Technology:** Apps and digital tools for relationship management can simplify tracking your TRACE metrics and progress. There are many apps designed to assist with goal setting, journaling, and time tracking, all of which can help you keep a record of the time and energy you invest in specific interactions. Some apps offer reminders and prompts to reflect on your goals and experiences, allowing for a consistent focus on improvement. With digital tools, you can set reminders, journal about your interactions, and observe your emotional awareness, helping to keep your TRACE metrics in view.

By incorporating these resources into your relationship journey, you'll find reliable methods to support and measure your efforts. Whether through professional guidance, educational environments, or practical digital aids, you'll be better equipped to manage TRACE metrics effectively, ultimately fostering healthier, more fulfilling relationships.

* * *

In this chapter, we explored how to use HEART and TRACE to shape healthier relationships grounded in your core values and beliefs. By applying the TRACE system—Time, Resistance, Awareness, Control, and Evolving—you've learned ways to approach your relationships with intention. This process includes self-reflection and the flow characteristics (clarity, centering, commitment, continuous feedback, challenge, and choice), each of which can foster progress in your relationships.

Reflecting on your relationships is more than examining your interactions; it involves assessing how you see yourself, others, and your broader world. By becoming intentional and embracing change, you lay the groundwork for relationships that align with your framework, and you deepen your connections with yourself and others.

In the next chapter, we'll apply the principles of Recreation and Recovery to TRACE, delving into how to cultivate downtime that not only rejuvenates but also sparks excitement in your life, time and time again. As you continue, remember that every step, whether in work or leisure, contributes to a balanced, meaningful life that aligns with your core values. Every action you take brings you closer to a life enriched by the designs you've imagined.

Pause and Reflect

Some reflection questions to help you on your relationship journey:

- How can you apply the autotelic personality traits (clarity, centering, commitment, continuous feedback, challenge, and choice) to foster positive changes in your relationships?
- Reflect on your self-perception across the past, present, and future. What shifts, if any, would improve your relationships?
- In what ways can you bring greater intentionality to your relationships with yourself, others, and the world around you?
- Are you planning to utilize resources such as counseling, classes, or technology to track your TRACE metrics and strengthen your relationships? How might these tools benefit you?
- What challenges might arise in applying TRACE metrics to relationships?
- How has your upbringing negatively affected your adult relationships?
- How has your upbringing positively affected your adult relationships?

CHAPTER 10

Prioritizing Recreation and Recovery

"The intellect must not be kept at consistent tension, but diverted by pastimes. [. . .] The mind must have relaxation, and will rise stronger and keener after recreation."[24]

—SENECA THE YOUNGER

I t's time to continue our exploration of HEART and TRACE with a focus on play, recreation, and recovery. When crafting a life of purpose, one must include purposeful relaxation, playfulness, and fun, as these play a vital role in finding balance in a holistic lifestyle. It's important to recognize that creative outlets, recreation, and recovery are critical to your overall health and well-being, including a combination of physical and mental stimulation and rest. Designing a life that incorporates these elements helps you foster a

---

24 Seneca the Younger, The Stoic Philosophy of Seneca: Essays and Letters, ed. Moses Hadas (W.W. Norton, 1968), 104.

deeper connection to yourself—remember the concept of *Self within Self*—and the world around you.

By bringing recreation and recovery into your journey, you're inviting a fuller connection to yourself, your creativity, and your ability to handle life's challenges with renewed energy. As you move through this chapter, consider how the autotelic traits—Clarity, Centeredness, Commitment, Continuous Feedback, Challenge, and Choice—can guide you in shaping a balanced and fulfilling approach to downtime. Each characteristic serves to remind you that these moments of relaxation and play aren't indulgences; they're building blocks for a life that sustains you, inspires you, and connects you to the world in meaningful ways.

In this chapter, we'll explore:

- **Recreation:** Activities that invigorate and inspire, cultivating joy, playfulness, and connection with oneself, others, and nature.

- **Recovery:** Practices that restore physical, mental, and emotional well-being, promoting balance and resilience.

- **Creative Expression:** Imaginative endeavors that broaden perspective, enhance self-awareness, and provide fulfillment through meaningful creation.

Let's dive into what regenerative recreation and recovery look like, beginning with a thoughtful reflection on the ways you currently engage with relaxation, play, and creativity. Together, we'll create a system that ensures these essential parts of life contribute to a strong, resilient foundation.

Self-Reflect on Your Recreation and Recovery

Take a moment to examine the role of recreation and recovery in your life, starting as far back as your childhood. From an early age, we often learn how to play and rest through the people and environments around us. This is where the priorities within the HEART framework intersect—your caregivers' health, enterprise, relationships, and sense of purpose, along with your own, shape your attitudes, habits, and behaviors regarding recreation and recovery. Reflecting on these experiences helps you identify whether you were taught (or learned) how to cultivate a healthy relationship with recreation and recovery, either as solitary activities or ones shared with others. An unhealthy or neglected history in this area may limit your understanding and ability to engage in what truly constitutes regenerative recreation and recovery.

Reflecting on these influences provides a window into your values and whether they've translated into a lifestyle that prioritizes creativity, play, and rest.

In these simple acts of play, rest, and creativity, you can uncover new insights about yourself and your needs. Evaluating how you engage in downtime not only sheds light on your overall well-being but also helps you design a life that incorporates both joy and renewal.

Questions to Guide Your Reflection

1. Do you have a creative outlet?

Think about how you express your creativity. Have you consistently engaged in creative pursuits since childhood, or did responsibilities, routines, or other challenges crowd them out? Some individuals struggle to connect with others because they were discouraged from play by authoritarian or overprotective parents, or because their caregivers lacked the resources to support recreational activities. These early experiences often have lasting consequences.

Consider what activities ignite your imagination and energize your mind. Do your creative pursuits evoke emotions and provide a meaningful escape? Creativity isn't just about producing something tangible; it enhances sensory awareness, fosters lateral thinking, and strengthens neural pathways in the brain.

2. Do you make time for play?

Playful activities, whether structured (e.g., team sports) or unstructured (e.g., spontaneous games), stimulate the mind and uplift the spirit. Play refreshes both the heart and mind, encouraging engagement and joy. It reminds us that delight can be found in even the simplest things. Reflect on moments when you prioritized play. How did those experiences make you feel? How often do you allow yourself this kind of carefree amusement today?

3. Are you getting adequate recreation and recovery?

Examine whether your current strategies for recreation and recovery meet your needs. Is your work–life–rest balance sustainable?

Pay attention to sleep patterns and daily habits, such as winding down before bed or creating a sleep-friendly environment. Are you sacrificing quality rest to accommodate other demands? Awareness of your rest habits can help you uncover ways to integrate more meaningful recovery time into your routine.

As you reflect on your childhood and current experiences, remember that recreation and recovery are complementary. Physical activities can be deeply relaxing, while creative and restful pursuits can be both stimulating and calming. Together, these forms of rejuvenation contribute to a holistic, leisure-filled life.

Identify Areas for Potential Change

As you work toward a life of intention, reflect on how your approach to recreation and recovery might benefit from a refresh. Recreation should energize and inspire, while recovery should genuinely restore. Begin by identifying routines that may have become habitual but no longer bring joy or rejuvenation. It's natural for your needs and preferences to evolve, and these changes offer an opportunity to reassess and realign.

Consider the balance among three key components: recreation, recovery, and creative expression. Do any of these areas feel overlooked? If your creative side has been dormant or if playfulness has taken a back seat to other priorities, this may be the moment to rediscover them. Similarly, evaluate whether your recovery habits truly support your physical and mental health. An imbalance in these areas may signal the need for change.

Indicators of a Need for Change

- **Routine Fatigue:** Recreational activities that once felt refreshing now feel monotonous or unfulfilling.

- **Quality and Quantity:** The frequency and nature of your recreation negatively impact your HEART priorities and disrupt your TRACE processes, resulting in unintended and natural consequences.

- **Lack of Joy:** Activities that once brought you pleasure now feel dull, obligatory, or mechanical.

- **Stress Accumulation:** Current recovery practices fail to alleviate stress, leaving you feeling persistently tense or fatigued.

Areas to Reevaluate

- **Time Allocation:** Reflect on how much intentional time you dedicate to creativity, play, and rest. Are you allocating enough time to these areas, or could adjustments be made to prioritize them?

- **Adaptability:** Consider whether your habits are flexible enough to accommodate changing circumstances or new interests. Are you open to exploring fresh activities that align with your evolving needs?

- **External Influences:** Identify external factors, such as work demands, social obligations, or environmental constraints, that may hinder your ability to fully engage in recreation or recovery. Adjusting boundaries or routines can help prioritize these activities.

By addressing these questions, you will pinpoint areas for small adjustments and, in some cases, a complete reset. Embracing these changes sets the stage for a more balanced and refreshing approach to downtime, one that fosters levity, renewal, and a vibrant sense of well-being.

Creating a Framework for Your Recreation and Recovery Objective

Imagine your ideal state of recreation and recovery. What does a balanced and fulfilling engagement in creativity, play, and rest look like for you? Consider the purpose these activities serve in your life, whether it's fostering joy, strengthening social connections, promoting personal growth, or enhancing overall well-being. Defining this purpose creates a foundation for recreation that is both rewarding and restorative.

As you craft your objectives in the realm of recreation, focus on aligning your pursuits with your core values and broader life vision. When recreation and recovery resonate with what matters most to you, they transform mere "time off" into an integral component of a purposeful lifestyle.

Impact of Recreation and Recovery on Health

Engaging in rest and creative activities nurtures both physical and mental well-being.

- **Benefits:** Restorative activities enhance cognitive function, reduce stress, and improve overall health.

- **Consequences of Neglect:** Failure to rest leads to stress buildup, exhaustion, and a weakened immune system.

- **Opportunity Costs:** Ignoring recovery fosters burnout, compromising long-term health and vitality.

- **Short- vs. Long-term Impact:** While skipping recovery may boost immediate productivity, over time it depletes both health and performance capacity.

Impact of Recreation and Recovery on Enterprise

Rest and creative outlets elevate productivity and decision-making.

- **Benefits:** Rested individuals are more creative, make better decisions, and experience greater job satisfaction.

- **Consequences of Neglect:** Overworking leads to burnout, poor decision-making, and cognitive fatigue.

- **Opportunity Costs:** Focusing solely on work at the expense of recovery limits professional growth and long-term effectiveness.

- **Short- vs. Long-term Impact:** While short-term overwork may seem efficient, prolonged neglect of recovery will result in burnout and stagnation.

Impact of Recreation and Recovery on Authentic Relationships

Shared rest and recreation deepen connections and enhance joy.

- **Benefits:** Collaborative leisure activities strengthen emotional bonds, reduce stress, and foster meaningful relationships.

- **Consequences of Neglect:** Neglecting quality time together weakens emotional ties and breeds isolation.

- **Opportunity Costs:** Prioritizing obligations over recreation degrades the quality and fulfillment of relationships.

- **Short- vs. Long-term Impact:** Neglecting shared time may feel productive in the short term, but over time it erodes relational health and satisfaction.

Impact of Recreation and Recovery on Transcendent Purpose and Meaning

Rest and creative expression provide space for introspection and alignment with deeper purpose.

- **Benefits:** Regular recovery fosters self-awareness, personal insight, and greater alignment with purpose.

- **Consequences of Neglect:** A life devoid of meaningful rest and play leads to burnout, stifling spiritual and personal development.

- **Opportunity Costs:** Neglecting rest hinders engagement with higher aspirations and impedes self-actualization.

- **Short- vs. Long-term Impact:** Constant action may feel purposeful in the short term, but neglecting rest ultimately disengages us from our true purpose and meaning.

Attach Your TRACE Metrics

Once you've established your recreation priorities, apply TRACE to make your goal measurable, actionable, and sustainable. Remember that the HEART framework is constantly intersecting but not mutually exclusive, i.e., the state of our health, enterprise, or relationships can affect the quality of recreation and recovery. However, recreation and recovery can be tailored to suit your specific needs. Below, we'll explore how specific processes can enhance recreation and relaxation. Here's how TRACE can help you structure and achieve this goal:

Time

Always set a realistic timeframe for your recreational, relaxing, or creative pursuits. Life visions shouldn't be left to chance or vague promises of "one of these days." Committing to a set time sharpens clarity and builds confidence, self-respect, and consistency, all key elements in skill development. When you view time as an investment in your well-being, you create a rhythm that nurtures both growth and enjoyment. Without a plan to invest time in recreation and recovery, a dream of the future quickly fades into a memory of the past, leaving you stuck in the pseudo-play of low-frequency "fun" or scrolling through social media. Such fleeting distractions and superficial engagement offer little more than empty satisfaction, leaving you more disconnected and thinking wishfully about what might have been.

Resistance

Learning any new skill comes with challenges, and hobbies, creativity, and rest are no exception. Identify potential sources of resistance, such as procrastination, daily responsibilities, or fatigue, and plan ahead to strategize around them. Approach avoidance and procrastination with a growth mindset, focusing on the long-term benefits and the new narratives that emerge from confronting resistance. Consider starting your day with a script for the ideal version of yourself—this sets the right tone for adopting new routines.

Awareness

Cultivate self-awareness by tracking your creative outlets and noting how they make you feel. Are you able to experience a flow state when engaged in these activities? Do the stories that emerge align with your ideal vision of yourself? Are these activities aligned with your authentic self? Do they deepen your connection with yourself, others, or nature, depending on your values? Are these activities rejuvenating and restorative? Regular reflection will help you assess what's working well and where adjustments are needed, keeping you engaged and motivated to continue growing.

Control

Exercise conscious control over your recreational, relaxation, and creative journey by setting specific milestones and breaking tasks down into manageable steps. Set boundaries to ensure these activities remain a consistent priority.

Flexibility in adapting to changes and challenges will make the process more enjoyable while keeping you focused on your vision.

Evolving

Establishing a creative and restorative routine is a process that requires ongoing adjustments. As you pursue this priority, you may find that changes are needed in several of your HEART priorities and TRACE processes to fully optimize it. Stay open to modifying your approach, seeking feedback, and exploring new methods of engagement. Embrace the inherent challenge and growth that come with skill acquisition, always keeping the larger benefits, joy, relaxation, and self-expression, in mind.

Applying TRACE in this way turns your recreation and recovery goal into an actionable plan, providing structure for your learning process and ensuring it remains aligned with your broader vision. When each metric of TRACE is thoughtfully applied, you deepen your experience, engage meaningfully, and cultivate excitement and confidence in your ability to master a new skill.

Integrating Technology into Recreation and Recovery

Technology offers access to tools that can enhance creativity, relaxation, learning, and overall well-being. By selecting tech tools that align with your goals, you can bring greater intention and variety to your free time, making recreation and recovery more impactful and fulfilling. Here are some ideas for mindfully incorporating technology into this area of your life:

- **Creativity Apps:** Digital platforms can provide new avenues for creative expression. Apps such as Procreate for digital art, Adobe Spark for graphic design, or GarageBand for music creation open up avenues to experiment and express yourself. Whether you're sketching, designing, or making music, these apps provide a satisfying sense of accomplishment that comes from creating something uniquely yours.

- **Rest and Relaxation Apps:** Apps that promote relaxation and stress reduction are invaluable for healthy recovery. Meditation apps such as Headspace and Calm offer guided mindfulness practices, deep breathing exercises, and peaceful visuals that help you unwind. White noise and ambient sound apps such as Rain Rain Sleep Sounds and Relax Melodies can support a restful sleep environment, helping you recharge and prepare for the day ahead.

- **Leisure and Entertainment Apps:** Leisure apps help bring joy to your downtime. Apps such as Amazon Kindle for e-books, Google Arts & Culture for virtual museum tours, or Spotify for music and podcasts open doors to immersive experiences. Enjoying high-quality leisure activities lets you tap into entertainment that aligns with your interests and values, enhancing your downtime.

- **Sleep Tracking Apps:** Quality sleep is essential for full recovery. Sleep tracking apps such as Sleep Cycle, Oura, Ultrahuman and Whoop, or devices such as Fitbit help monitor your sleep patterns, providing insights on sleep quality and recommending adjustments for improvement. A well-rested body and mind are key to sustaining your well-being and preparing you for a productive day.

- **Mindfulness Apps:** Apps dedicated to mindfulness can foster mental clarity and reduce stress. Options such as Pacifica for anxiety management, Breathwrk for guided breathing exercises, or Simple Habit for quick meditation sessions help integrate relaxation into your routine, creating moments of calm amidst daily demands.

When used intentionally, technology can be a valuable companion in your recreation and recovery journey, enhancing activities in ways that align with your personal goals. These tools promote engagement in meaningful pursuits, supporting well-being and adding richness to your recreation and recovery. Take a moment to reflect on which apps or tools might add value to your routine, and consider how they might enhance your pursuit of a life worth living.

* * *

As you continue framing your life with intention, it's essential to recognize the significance of recreation and recovery. These are not merely pleasant additions to your schedule; they are crucial components of a balanced, fulfilling life. They offer an opportunity to reconnect with a sense of playfulness, engage your inner child, reduce stress, and recharge your mind, body, and spirit. By prioritizing these restorative activities, you're strengthening the foundation that enables you to face challenges with resilience, creativity, and purpose.

Reflecting on how you spend your free time helps you discover what truly rejuvenates you, bringing clarity to what makes recreation meaningful in your life. Purposeful recreation and recovery, whether through play, creative expression, or mindful relaxation, allow you to reconnect with yourself and replenish the physical and mental reserves needed to live with vitality.

Recreation and recovery are not luxuries but essential tools for well-being. When you fully understand their role, you're better equipped to prioritize and integrate them into your life intentionally. This balance is key to crafting a life worth living, one that's not only productive but deeply satisfying.

In the final chapter of this section, we'll bring together everything you've reflected on so far as you begin integrating your purpose into the system. Together, we'll take the next step toward shaping a life aligned with your core values, one that reflects your most authentic self and brings fulfillment through a harmonious blend of work, play, and rest.

Pause and Reflect

Here are some reflection questions to help you on your HEART journey:

- What creative outlets make you feel energized and fulfilled? How can you incorporate more of these activities into your daily routine?
- How can you intentionally infuse moments of play into your day to reduce stress and enhance overall well-being?
- Evaluate your current strategies for recreation and recovery. What effective activities have you consistently engaged in to foster healthy play, creativity, and recovery?
- Without judgment, what habits have you turned to as a means of relaxation and play that have been unhealthy and ineffective?
- Have you explored apps that can enhance your creativity, improve sleep, or support your learning and leisure pursuits?
- How can you integrate technology mindfully to complement your well-being?
- How can you design your life to regularly incorporate a dedicated day or span of days on which you do absolutely nothing?

CHAPTER 11

Transcendent Purpose and Meaning

"Life is never made unbearable by circumstances,
but only by lack of meaning and purpose."[25]

—VIKTOR FRANKL

A s we reach the final chapter of this section, it's time to connect the dots among the five facets of HEART. We've delved into Health, Enterprise, Authentic Relationships, and Recreation and Recovery and how each helps building a meaningful life. Now, we bring them together to uncover the essence of Transcendent Purpose and Meaning—the anchor that ties your life to something greater than the ordinary.

––––––––––––

25   Viktor Frankl Zentrum Wien (@franklzentrum), "Quote of the Week by Viktor E. Frankl," Facebook, June 27, 2024, https://www.facebook.com/ share/p/19Fv2VL8MA/.

Transcendent Purpose and Meaning is your call to self-actualization. It is the guiding thread of purpose that shapes your days, the narrative you're writing with every choice. To live with open-eyed intention, you must reflect on what drives you, align your actions with that deeper story, and transform your potential into kinetic energy through unwavering commitment to what truly matters to you.

This elevates your life experience to something of great importance. This approach to transcendence means your health, relationships, work, recreation, and rest require your presence and participation from moment to moment. It means your health and all the things you do to replenish your body and mind are of the utmost importance and an investment in not only your present self but your future self and all others who will come to need you to be healthy for them. It means your relationships should not be taken for granted, and it requires your best self to show up every day and to implement boundaries to protect what you have built. With this attitude in mind, we come to realize moments and opportunities we may have underappreciated or overlooked. This also gives us easy access to experiences of gratitude for the moments when we still have to adapt.

If you want to build a life worth living, identifying your purpose and shaping the story you want your life to tell are essential. This requires peak self-awareness, a willingness to examine your values, motivations, and goals with honesty and intentionality. In the pages ahead, we'll explore practical ways to prioritize your purpose and meaning, ensuring they become effective and achievable parts of your daily life.

Transcendent Purpose and Meaning is comprised of three core elements:

- **Self-Actualization and Fulfillment:** The pursuit of your highest potential, living authentically and embracing the fullness of who you are.

- **Purpose:** A clear and guiding sense of why you do what you do; the deeper motivation that fuels your every action.

- **The Narrative or Story:** The life you are crafting with every choice, where each chapter weaves your decisions into a legacy that stretches beyond the fleeting moment.

Self-Reflect on Your Life's Purpose and Meaning

Self-reflection here is an introspective journey where awareness plays a vital role. This process entails deep contemplation on the desired impact on your life and how it ripples through others. It involves understanding personal values, experiences, ideals, and beliefs, maybe more so than all the other facets of HEART priorities. Indeed, your purpose and the story you want to tell or have told about your life will drive all those other segments of your life worth living. Purpose and meaning become the guide that shapes the rest and empowers us to adapt and release all other unproductive priorities.

There are many ways that you can take deliberate time to self-reflect on your purpose. Although we've already touched on a few in previous chapters, look at this list and see which ones you think would work well with your personality and proclivities.

- **Journaling:** Dedicate time to write about your values, aspirations, and the impact you want to have on yourself and others. Reflect on moments of fulfillment and what brings you joy. What story are you currently telling with your life? Are the highs and lows contributing to a meaningful narrative, or does the story need rewriting? Have you inherited a script from those before you, carrying on patterns that no longer serve you?

- **Mindfulness and Meditation:** Engage in mindfulness practices to cultivate awareness of your body, mind, and emotions in the present moment. By observing without judgment, you gain clarity on how these elements influence your choices and align with your values. Meditation offers a space to connect with your inner self and explore your relationship with the outer world. Through stillness and focused attention, you gain a deeper understanding of your purpose, allowing you to uncover what truly matters and how you wish to contribute to the world.

- **Life Mapping:** Create a visual representation of your life, highlighting significant events, achievements, and moments of growth. This can help identify patterns and themes that point toward your purpose.

- **Talking to Mentors or Trusted Friends:** Seek guidance and feedback from mentors or people you trust. Discussing your aspirations with others can provide valuable insights and perspectives.

- **Values Assessment:** Identify your core values and assess how well your current actions align with them. Adjustments can be made to ensure your life is in harmony with your fundamental beliefs.

- **Vision Board:** Create a vision board that represents your goals and desires. Display it in a visible place to serve as a daily reminder of your purpose.

- **Reading and Learning:** Explore books and other media focused on philosophy, or attend workshops that explore the concept of purpose and meaning. Learning from experts and the experiences of others can offer valuable insights.

- **Feedback and Self-Reflection:** Solicit feedback from peers, colleagues, or friends about your strengths and areas of impact. Combine this external perspective with self-reflection to refine your understanding of your purpose.

- **Nature and Solitude:** Spend time in nature or engage in activities that allow for solitude. The rawness of a natural environment can facilitate introspection and provide clarity about your purpose and your life's story.

These activities can help you incorporate self-reflection into your life as a continuous process. Making a habit of cultivating self-awareness is a tremendous way to ensure that you are always seeking to stay on target to live a life worth living.

Identify Areas of Potential Change

When framing your purpose and meaning, you must deeply understand the areas in your life that are begging for transformation. Identifying these spaces where change is not only possible but necessary is a vital step in aligning your actions with the goal of a life worth living. The significance of this process becomes apparent when we consider the interconnected nature of your HEART priorities. Here are some things to consider when trying to determine your purpose using the self-reflection methods listed above.

Core Values

- **Reflective Step:** Take time to reflect on your core values and assess whether your current pursuits align with them. Are there areas of your life where your actions contradict your beliefs? Do you follow through on what matters most to you, or are there misalignments that need addressing? Identifying these gaps can offer valuable insights and reveal areas ripe for transformation.

- **Why It Matters:** Your core values act as the compass that directs your decisions and actions. They are the silent architects behind the life you lead and the choices you make. When your pursuits stray from these foundational values, misalignment results, sparking inner conflict and steering you away from a life that reflects your true self. This deviation can shape an alternate history, one where fulfillment and purpose are compromised. Identifying and addressing these misalignments are essential steps for recalibrating your journey toward a life of authenticity, ensuring that each action is in harmony with your deeper purpose.

Personal Growth Assessment

- **Reflective Step:** Evaluate your journey of personal growth with a wide lens. Identify the thoughts, actions, and habits that have fueled your most significant progress as well as those that have left you feeling stagnant or unfulfilled. Pinpointing these areas can highlight the need for change and further development.

- **Why It Matters:** Personal growth is influenced by ongoing internal and external processes integral to purposeful living. Stagnation in certain aspects of your life can impede the overall fulfillment of your purpose. Recognizing these areas allows you to target them for adjustment and transformation.

Impact on Others

- **Reflective Step:** Consider the impact your narratives, actions, and choices have on others. Are your pursuits positively contributing a positive chapter to the book of the lives of those around you? What stories do you want others to tell about you? Identifying areas where your impact can be enhanced creates an atmosphere of meaningful connections.

- **Why It Matters:** Purpose often transcends the individual and involves a communal element. Understanding your influence on others enables you to create a ripple effect of positivity and meaning. This reflection empowers you to align your actions with the values and legacy you want to embody.

Clarify Your Contribution

- **Reflective Step:** Assess the clarity of your unique contribution to your community and the world. Do your skills and passions align with solving broader challenges? Identifying ambiguity in your understanding of this connection opens opportunities to sharpen your focus and amplify your impact.

- **Why It Matters:** Clarity in your contribution enhances the effectiveness and significance of your efforts. When you align your passions and skills with purposeful action, you maximize your ability to leave a lasting mark on others and the world. Recognizing and addressing gaps in clarity ensures your contributions are both meaningful and impactful.

Leaving a Legacy

- **Reflective Step:** Envision the legacy you wish to leave behind. What kind of impact do you want to make, and how do you want to be remembered? Reflect on the stories that might be told about you by loved ones and the broader world. Identifying alignment or conflicts with this vision helps you clarify and pursue a purpose-driven legacy.

- **Why It Matters:** Deliberately shaping your legacy enables you to live with intention and influence. Reflecting on how your current pursuits align with your vision for the future provides direction, ensuring that your choices today contribute meaningfully to the story you want to leave behind.

You lay the path to a purpose-driven life by aligning your core values, assessing your growth, evaluating your impact on others, reflecting on your desired legacy, and clarifying your contribution. This intentional self-reflection empowers you to make choices that resonate with your values. You will grow, create meaningful contributions, and leave a legacy that inspires others. This is authentic living.

Creating a Framework for Your Transcendent Purpose Objective

Crafting a framework for transcendent purpose and meaning involves outlining a clear and inspiring direction that aligns with your core values, leverages your strengths, and resonates with your vision of a meaningful life. As you map out this transformation, consider setting objectives that embody the following aspects:

Impact of Transcendent Purpose and Meaning on Health

A clear sense of purpose supports physical, mental, and spiritual resilience.

- **Benefits:** A life driven by purpose provides the motivation to care for one's body and mind, fostering well-being through alignment with values and goals. Spiritual alignment with purpose creates a deep sense of peace and fulfillment, enhancing emotional health.

- **Consequences of Neglect:** Without purpose, physical and mental health deteriorate as the drive to care for oneself diminishes. Spiritual emptiness results in confusion and existential stress, harming overall well-being.

- **Opportunity Costs:** A lack of purpose leads to emotional exhaustion and health decline as individuals struggle to find meaning in their daily lives.

- **Short- vs. Long-term Impact:** In the short term, a lack of purpose may seem manageable, but over time it creates physical and mental strain, limiting one's ability to fully engage with life's potential.

Impact of Transcendent Purpose and Meaning on Enterprise

Aligning one's work with one's deeper values fuels professional success and satisfaction.

- **Benefits:** Living with purpose imbues work with meaning, fostering intrinsic motivation and satisfaction. When aligned with a life narrative, work becomes more than a job; it becomes a contribution to something greater.

- **Consequences of Neglect:** Without purpose, work becomes a series of monotonous tasks that drain energy and satisfaction, leading to burnout and disengagement.

- **Opportunity Costs:** Focusing solely on external rewards without connecting to a deeper sense of purpose leads to unfulfilling success and missed opportunities for meaningful contributions.

- **Short- vs. Long-term Impact:** Short-term financial gain might bring temporary satisfaction, but over time, a life without purpose leaves individuals feeling empty, disconnected, and unfulfilled in their careers.

Impact of Transcendent Purpose and Meaning on Authentic Relationships

A clear sense of purpose strengthens relationships, providing a shared sense of meaning and promoting gratitude for the valuable relationships we have with ourselves, others, and the natural world.

- **Benefits:** Shared values and purpose foster deeper emotional connections, creating a sense of mutual growth and alignment in relationships. Spiritual purpose unites individuals in their pursuit of a greater good, enriching relationships with love and mutual understanding.

- **Consequences of Neglect:** Without purpose, relationships become shallow and strained as individuals struggle to find meaning in their interactions.

- **Opportunity Costs:** Failing to cultivate a shared life narrative weakens relational bonds and makes relationships feel unfulfilling and emotionally barren.

- **Short- vs. Long-term Impact:** While casual relationships may provide temporary satisfaction, over time, relationships rooted in shared purpose and a unified narrative offer deeper fulfillment and lasting emotional connection.

Impact of Transcendent Purpose and Meaning on Recreation and Recovery

Purposeful recreation supports personal growth, reflection, and the alignment of life's goals.

- **Benefits:** Recreation aligned with purpose provides opportunities for self-discovery, introspection, and renewal. Spiritual practices integrated into leisure activities foster a deeper connection to one's purpose.

- **Consequences of Neglect:** Recreation without meaning becomes hollow, offering no real recovery or emotional enrichment.

- **Opportunity Costs:** Prioritizing mindless distractions over intentional recreation prevents access to creative insight and growth, leaving individuals disconnected from themselves and their potential.

- **Short- vs. Long-term Impact:** Short-term, mindless recreation may provide temporary relief, but long-term investment in practicing adaptive play and creativity fosters personal growth, neuroplasticity, and alignment with one's life narrative.

Attach Your TRACE Metrics

Here's how to apply TRACE metrics to your life goals to build a life worth living:

Time

Time represents the finite yet profound resource through which we align our behaviors with our values and long-term vision. Purpose, by its nature, often transcends temporal boundaries, creating a paradox where we need to use limited moments to create a lasting legacy. By prioritizing intentional, meaningful activities over transient or trivial pursuits, we contribute to a life story that is both purposeful and enduring. Actionable steps include conducting weekly, monthly, quarterly, and yearly time audits to assess how current activities reflect personal priorities and creating a schedule that dedicates time to activities that align with one's long-term goals, such as volunteering, deep learning, or creative expression.

Resistance

While time provides the framework for purposeful action, resistance often challenges our ability to remain aligned with our goals. Resistance, both internal and external, is a natural obstacle in the pursuit of purpose. Internally, resistance may manifest as self-doubt or fear of failure, while externally, it can stem from societal pressures or systemic limitations. Overcoming resistance requires both awareness and strategic action. Actionable steps include reframing negative self-talk into constructive narratives, seeking allies and mentorship to navigate external challenges, and engaging in practices such as cognitive-restructuring techniques or mindfulness to address internal resistance.

Awareness

Overcoming resistance requires clarity, which is cultivated through self-awareness and understanding of our environment. Insight, or self-awareness, helps us identify our intrinsic motivations, values, and sources of fulfillment, while outsight, or external awareness, helps us situate our purpose within the context of broader societal needs. Actionable steps include engaging in reflective journaling to clarify personal values and periodically conducting a "purpose alignment check" to evaluate whether current activities resonate with overarching goals. Additionally, engaging in deep learning about the world, such as exploring global issues or gaining cross-disciplinary insights through dialogue with others or participating in community initiatives, can deepen internal and external awareness.

Control

Awareness provides the insights necessary to exercise control, enabling us to take deliberate action toward purposeful goals. Control focuses on exercising our autonomy over aspects of life that align with our purpose while maintaining adaptability in the face of unpredictability (i.e., negentropy vs entropy). Developing a sense of control involves recognizing areas within one's influence and optimizing them. Actionable steps include setting SMART (Specific, Measurable, Achievable, Relevant, and Time-bound) goals for purposeful activities and identifying contingency plans for anticipated obstacles to maintain progress even during disruptions.

Evolving

As we establish control, the need to adapt and evolve ensures our purpose remains aligned with the ever-changing landscape of life. This emphasizes the dynamic nature of purpose, encouraging individuals to embrace growth and change as their understanding of meaning shifts over time. Purpose is not fixed but evolves through the integration of new experiences and challenges. Actionable steps may include scheduling quarterly reflections to review significant life events and their impact on one's larger personal purpose, setting aside time for exploratory learning, and updating personal narratives to incorporate evolving goals and values.

TRACE metrics serve as a model for a strategic framework. By regularly reflecting on and adapting the TRACE framework, you can ensure your strategies remain flexible and dynamic, enabling you to navigate challenges and make a sustained, meaningful impact on your world.

* * *

As we conclude the exploration of purpose and meaning, you should by now recognize that aligning your life's purpose with HEART priorities is not just a theoretical exercise but a transformative journey. Reflecting on the life story you're creating, identifying areas for change, creating HEART objectives, and tracking your progress with TRACE metrics are steps toward living a life imbued with meaning and intentionality.

Now it's time for us to head into Part Three, where we'll synthesize the five facets of HEART into a practical, unified road map, equipping you with tools and practices to harmonize your priorities and unlock your highest potential. Together, we'll explore strategies to integrate these principles into every facet of your life for holistic, meaningful growth.

Pause and Reflect

Some reflection questions to help you on your Purpose journey:

- How does your current life's purpose align with your values and the other four facets of HEART—health, enterprise, authentic relationships, and recreation and recovery?
- Reflect on instances when a lack of alignment between your purpose and your life's story led to inner conflict or feelings of disconnection. How might realigning these aspects with your purpose bring greater fulfillment?
- Are there areas in your life where you feel your life's story isn't fully integrated? For instance, do career goals sometimes clash with personal relationships, or does recreation feel overshadowed by enterprise? How could recalibrating these areas strengthen your overall sense of purpose?
- Reflect on the progress you've made in pursuing your purpose and meaning. What TRACE metrics could you implement to track this progress more effectively? For example, you might measure time spent on meaningful pursuits, evaluate the quality of your relationships, or assess how intentional choices have shaped your health or creativity.
- How might aligning your purpose with other HEART priorities positively impact your overall well-being and sense of fulfillment? Consider the ripple effects, such as how improved health might energize your enterprise or how authentic relationships might deepen your sense of purpose.

PART THREE

Putting It All Together

CHAPTER 12

Finding Flow

"We are what we repeatedly do. Excellence, then, is not an act, but a habit."[26]

—WILL DURANT

O ver the last several chapters, we've extensively explored each aspect of the HEART framework, Health, Authentic Relationships, Enterprise, Recreation and Recovery, and Transcendent Purpose and Meaning, and we've examined how each of these priorities contributes to a dynamic, adventurous life that transcends mere surviving. We've also examined the traits of an autotelic personality, Clarity, Centeredness, Commitment, Continuous Feedback, Challenge, and Choice. By delving into these interconnected aspects of life, we've created objectives for each HEART priority and attached TRACE processes (Time, Resistance, Awareness, Control, and Evolving) to achieve those goals.

---

26 Will Durant, The Story of Philosophy: The Lives and Opinions of the World's Greatest Philosophers (1926), Chapter II, Part VII.

In this chapter, we will focus on adopting and implementing a sense of flow, those optimal conditions where time seems to stand still and life becomes an immersive adventure in our newly developed operating system. We'll explore practical ways to integrate your HEART priorities and TRACE processes into a cohesive framework for creating a life worth living.

As discussed, the HEART priorities are not isolated; they are deeply interconnected. Building a cohesive framework means finding harmony and alignment between these moving parts. That may sound complex, but the examples below demonstrate how these systems can be customized to fit individual needs. As you examine your goals, you'll find substantial overlap, and many objectives can serve multiple purposes.

Let's dive in.

Identifying Overlapping and Standalone Objectives

Although everyone's goals will vary, examining examples can help clarify the concept. Since five seems to be our magic number, here are five examples of HEART goals that serve single and dual purposes:

Example 1: Mindful Eating

- **Overlapping Objectives:** Cultivating mindful eating habits enhances physical health and fosters deeper connections through shared meals, improving relationships.

- **Standalone Objective:** Running a marathon is a personal fitness goal that targets physical health without direct overlap with other priorities.

Example 2: Professional Development

- **Overlapping Objectives:** Pursuing an entrepreneurial path aligned with your values can both advance your career and enhance your personal sense of purpose.

- **Standalone Objective:** Attending workshops to enhance technical skills is a career-specific goal focused solely on professional development.

Example 3: Learning a New Language

- **Overlapping Objectives:** Learning a new language is both a recreational pursuit and an opportunity to connect with others in a way that enriches relationships.

- **Standalone Objective:** Traveling to a specific country for leisure is a goal within recreation and recovery, without direct overlap with relationships.

Example 4: Volunteer Leadership

- **Overlapping Objectives:** Taking on a leadership role in a volunteer organization nurtures relationships and also fulfills a larger purpose of contributing to a cause.

- **Standalone Objective:** Organizing a family reunion focuses on strengthening familial bonds and fits into the relationship priority.

Example 5: Meditation Practice

- **Overlapping Objectives:** A daily meditation practice supports mental health and also provides time for self-reflection, contributing to a sense of purpose.

- **Standalone Objective:** Participating in a fitness challenge focuses on physical health alone, without contributing directly to other priorities.

Not every goal has to serve more than one priority. However, pairing objectives stimulates lateral thinking and makes the time spent working toward them more productive. If you're striving for a holistic approach to your HEART priorities and their corresponding TRACE metrics, consider the following steps to consolidate your system.

Steps to Build Your Cohesive System

1. **Reflect on Your Values:** Assess your core values across your HEART priorities: health, enterprise, authentic relationships, recreation and recovery, and transcendent purpose and meaning. Identify areas where values overlap.

2. **Assess Your Current Goals:** Review your current aspirations and note common themes that span multiple priorities.

3. **Explore Interconnections:** Look for opportunities where achieving a goal in one priority positively impacts another.

4. **Consider Your Long-Term Vision:** Align your goals with your larger vision of fulfillment and purpose. Ensure each goal contributes to your overarching life story.

5. **Seek Feedback:** Discuss your goals with trusted individuals to uncover connections or areas of overlap that may not be immediately apparent.

6. **Evaluate Resource Utilization:** Consider how time, energy, and skills allocated to one goal may benefit another. Look for opportunities to optimize resource use.

7. **Embrace Flexibility:** Recognize that your priorities may evolve. Be open to adjusting your system as you grow.

8. **Align with Your Personal Mission:** Ensure your goals resonate with your personal mission and contribute to your sense of purpose.

9. **Prioritize Well-Being:** Choose goals that enhance your holistic health and happiness. Assess how each goal impacts your well-being.

10. **Conduct Periodic Reviews:** Regularly review your progress and refine your system as necessary to ensure continuous growth.

Let this list serve as a guide to constructing a cohesive framework by identifying both overlapping and standalone goals across your HEART priorities.

Consolidating Your Action Items

Once you've mapped out your goals, the next crucial step is to consolidate your action items. This involves not only setting clear tasks but also strategizing how personal resources can be efficiently allocated. By integrating your goals into a unified plan, you create a clear road map to achieve meaningful outcomes across your HEART priorities.

Practical Strategies for Implementation

Although we've discussed the concept of a life worth living in broad strokes, the reality is that we all have finite hours in a day and limited energy. The following strategies can help you make the most of your resources:

Time Management

- Prioritize tasks based on their alignment with your HEART priorities.
- Allocate blocks of focused time for each priority.
- Set realistic deadlines for specific objectives within each priority.

Adaptive Control

- Identify and protect the areas within each HEART priority where you have control.
- Focus on what you can influence, and adapt to factors that require flexibility.

- Practice radical acceptance, embracing the wisdom to know what is beyond your control and the clarity to focus on those things that are within your control.

Managing Change

- Anticipate changes and challenges within each priority.
- Create contingency plans for obstacles you may encounter.
- View change as a growth opportunity rather than a setback.

Handling Resistance

- Understand that resistance will arise across all HEART priorities.
- Break resistance down into manageable steps to target specific challenges.
- Seek support or guidance when necessary to overcome resistance effectively.

Sharpening Awareness

- Recognize patterns and cycles, both internal and external, that help or hinder your progress.
- Focus on what truly matters to you while minimizing distractions.
- Seek mentorship to learn from experts, bypass avoidable mistakes, and accelerate growth, all while leaving space for personal discovery.

Consolidating Personal Resources

Given that our time and energy are limited, consolidating resources to focus on what matters most is key to living a meaningful life. Here are strategies for optimizing your personal resources:

Time Resources

- Set aside specific time blocks for activities that serve multiple HEART priorities.

- Look for activities that influence multiple areas. For example, exercising with a friend enhances both your health and your relationships.

Energy Resources

- Allocate your energy based on the priority of goals within each HEART facet.
- Ensure proper recreation and recovery to maintain optimal energy levels.

Skill Resources

- Identify transferable skills that can be applied across different HEART priorities.
- Invest in skill development that boosts performance in multiple facets of life.

Emotional Resources

- Cultivate emotional resilience by recalling your wins and the difficulties you have overcome as you've navigated challenges in any HEART priority.
- Foster healthy emotional states through pleasurable activities that align with your personal goals.

Relational Resources

- Seek guidance from mentors, friends, and allies when needed.
- Build relationships with people who share your values, especially those with expertise that can help you grow.
- Leverage your allies as sentinels to scout out valuable opportunities, and offer your support to them in turn.

TRACE Your Steps

In the pursuit of a purposeful and harmonious life, *TRACE Your Steps* means integrating the principles of Time, Resistance, Awareness, Control, and Evolving (TRACE) across all HEART priorities. Thoughtfully managing your resources, time, energy, skills, and emotions, helps streamline your efforts and ensures steady progress toward your multifaceted objectives. This strategic approach not only enhances efficiency but also supports a balanced, integrated life. By cultivating this holistic approach, you can effectively manage overlapping and standalone goals while staying true to the principles of a life worth living.

Pause and Reflect

Some reflection questions to help you on your journey:

- How can you align your physical, mental, and spiritual practices to enhance your daily experiences across the HEART priorities? Reflect on how these foundational needs intersect with health, enterprise, relationships, recreation, and purpose, and explore ways to balance them seamlessly.

- In what ways can you nurture your relationships with both yourself and others to contribute to a more harmonious and fulfilling life? Consider strategies for deepening authenticity and connection, whether through active listening, quality time, or fostering a stronger bond with nature.

- What steps can you take to pursue your purpose and integrate it into your daily activities within the HEART framework? Identify actions, however small, that would align with your goals and values, enabling you to weave purpose into your everyday routines.

- How do you currently engage in meaningful leisure, and how can you optimize your leisure activities to achieve a state of flow within the context of the HEART priorities?

- Reflect on how your recreational activities rejuvenate you, and explore ways you can deepen your engagement for creative fulfillment.

- Reflect on the patterns or conditions that lead you to the flow state. How can you intentionally design your tasks and environments to support a flow state and enjoy a more engaging experience across the HEART priorities?

- How can you design intentional processes to focus your attention on what truly matters to you across all HEART priorities, eliminating the noise that detracts from meaningful pursuits?

CHAPTER 13

A Life Worth Living

*"The real self is not something one finds
as much as it is something one makes."*[27]

—SYDNEY J. HARRIS

W e've reached the final chapter in our journey together, where it is time to synthesize everything you've learned and consider your long-term outlook. How will the changes and adaptations you've made using HEART and TRACE impact your life now, a year from now, a decade from now? And what happens if mitigating circumstances put a damper on your plans? Let's recap what we know about priorities, processes, and autotelism while going over some contingency strategies for when things happen outside of your control.

----

27 . Sydney J. Harris, Strictly Personal (syndicated), Record-Gazette, Banning, California, April 18, 1969, page 10, https://www.newspapers.com/image/688575321/.

Holistic Harmony:
HEART, TRACE, and Autotelism

In Chapter 12, we looked at practical approaches to consolidating priorities and processes, helping you recognize where to prioritize and combine resources to achieve milestones. This includes everything from outlining your vision, goals, and schedules to adapting your mindset, emotion-set and behavior-set to creating a self-rewarding holistic system.

Sustain Your HEART Priorities

Despite the popular myth, building a habit isn't a 21-day challenge; it's a lived process, shaped by rhythm, repetition, and relationship with context. A study headed by behavioral psychologist Phillippa Lally showed that it takes an average of 66 days for a behavior to begin feeling automatic. For some, it's quicker; for others, it unfolds over several months.[28] Simpler habits integrate faster, while more complex shifts, like adopting a new fitness routine, require deeper consistency and care. A study of new gym members by Navin Kaushal and Ryan E. Rhodes found that even six weeks of regular engagement can begin to lay a foundation for a new exercise routine. The process is non-linear: progress often starts fast, then slows into a quiet settling. Importantly, missing a day doesn't erase the work.[29] In sum, habits don't form in days; they are cultivated over time, through intention and devotion.

More important than how long it takes to make or break a habit is the consistency required to create lasting, sustainable change. Why do we use the word *sustainable* when talking about change and goals? Because we want to ensure that our goals become part of an overall lifestyle inseparable from routines of daily living such as brushing one's teeth, taking a shower, or getting dressed for the day. We must think, act, and feel like the version of ourselves we want to be.

---

28   Lally et al., 2010.

29   Kaushal and Rhodes, 2015.

If you're struggling with any aspect of your HEART priorities, you can assess whether the problem is due to one or more of the five TRACE processes discussed in previous chapters. These processes and metrics provide us with the metacognitive awareness to make adjustments and regain control of our vision for our lives. One consequence of this attention to detail is adopting a way of being and an operating system that flows seamlessly.

On Gratitude, Radical Acceptance, Compassion, and Expectations (GRACE)

As you journey toward purpose, embrace the art of managing attachment to outcomes. In an ever-changing world, anything can happen, and the only aspect within your control is the quality of your response and effort. This underscores the significance of gratitude, radical acceptance, compassion, and managing expectations. Across health, enterprise, authentic relationships, recreation, and transcendent purpose and meaning, one constant remains: change. We exist in a liminal space between becoming and unbecoming, entropy and negentropy—between beginnings and endings—in a never-ending dance. Regardless of your pursuits and accomplishments, it is vital to acknowledge that nothing is promised. Gratitude, radical acceptance, compassion for self and others, managing expectations, and an understanding of life's mercurial nature are essential habits to cultivate.

Gratitude

Gratitude is the practice of acknowledging simple joys, ephemeral moments, and interconnectedness. They are there if you look closely enough. Gratitude allows you to savor the past, embrace the present, and anticipate the future, constructing a meaningful story even in the face of adversity. It is a transformative force that enriches both your life and the lives of those around you. Gratitude also reveals what often lingers unnoticed, quietly vital in the periphery of our awareness. Gratitude holds a profound place in creating a life worth living. By cultivating gratitude, you not only find solace amidst life's uncertainties but also gain a deeper appreciation for its intricacies.

Millions of people around the world face unforeseen tribulations despite their hard work, ethical fidelity, dedicated practices, and ascetic commitment to one belief or another. We expect to show up to a job and not receive a pink slip. We expect our partners and friends to continue playing their roles with blind admiration. We expect that our bodies will continue to hold up in spite of the rigors of the world and many of the things we put ourselves through. Yet life reminds us otherwise. We shudder at hearing the stories of people who were lucky (If you can call it that) enough to discover that nature had planted some genetic time bomb inside them that escaped detection until a routine checkup.

We expect the world and all its institutions to continue to function without interruption. Many of us can testify to the reality that things can turn helter-skelter in the blink of an eye. A pandemic. A war. A breakup. A divorce. An illness. An accident. A betrayal. That one mistake from years ago. A miscalculation. A misstep. You misspoke. You forgot. You remembered. You were too early. Too late. On time. Too fast. Too slow. On pace. The straw that broke the camel's back. The last drop of water that collapsed the levee. Why did it happen over there and not here? Why did it happen to them and not us? Why did it happen to him or her and not you, until you realize that one person's *there* is another person's *here*. One person's *them* is another person's *us*.

Maybe you're special. Maybe you are lucky. Maybe it's just not your turn—yet. Nothing is owed to us. Despite our surgical preparations, fate sometimes has other plans. Adopting this attitude fosters a climate of gratitude for even the most minuscule of blessings.

Gratitude becomes easier when we adopt the mindset that the universe does not inherently *owe* us anything—in essence, when we manage our conditioned personal and collective expectations of what the world is supposed to be like. With this attitude, we can appreciate life's subtleties and the smallest of experiences. By reframing our expectations, we can better appreciate life's subtleties: the breath filling our lungs, the cool breeze on our skin, the bed we sleep in, the companionship of those who care. The clean water we drink.

The privilege of knowing that the only nightmares you've had existed solely in your dreams and never outside your door. The roof over your head. The perceived failure that, in hindsight, led to opportunity. When we practice gratitude, the privileges we take for granted, such as safety and access to resources and opportunities, come into sharper focus.

Gratitude tunes us into the blessings we often overlook, redirecting our focus from what is missing to what is present.

The journey through HEART and TRACE demands intentionality and self-reflection on gratitude. Through this process comes the reconfiguration of beliefs, emotions, relationships, behaviors, and values that terraform the worldview that shapes your life. In this process, you begin to see that you, along with countless others and the forces of nature, are the catalysts behind the kinetic reshaping of your life. This awareness reveals countless reasons to be grateful, both within and beyond yourself.

Radical Acceptance

Practicing radical acceptance daily can alleviate intense suffering, reducing it to something more manageable, ordinary pain that every person experiences to some degree. Life's ordinary pains, stemming from the imperfections of being human in an imperfect world, are unavoidable. From the physical discomforts of the body to the psychological strains of the mind, life presents countless challenges that leave us dissatisfied, disappointed, blindsided, hurt, sad, deprived, surprised, angry, exhausted, or utterly fed up. In varying degrees, everyone encounters unfairness, injustice, chaos, confusion, and betrayal, sometimes despite their best efforts.

If we are fortunate, we can experience all these misfortunes without sinking into the hellscape of unnecessary and unrelenting suffering that stems from resisting reality. The key lies in seeing life for what it is.

So, what is radical acceptance? It is the ability to acknowledge life as it is, warts and all, without expecting it to be anything different in the moment. It doesn't mean we approve of or condone the situation, only that we recognize it and accept its reality at face value. Importantly, this isn't about giving up or acting helpless. It's about reframing our attitude and managing the expectation that life *must* be other than what it is.

A Practical Example

Imagine you're heading to an important interview and plan to arrive 30 minutes early, only to find yourself stuck in traffic due to an accident. You realize you'll now be 10 minutes late. What do you do? Naturally, frustration, irritability, and perhaps anger will arise—these are valid, ordinary pains that need to be acknowledged. But how does this escalate into suffering? Screaming out the window or honking your horn won't improve the situation. In fact, it might worsen it, causing both you and others additional suffering. Radical acceptance in this scenario means acknowledging the reality that there's no way to undo the traffic. Instead, you can explore alternatives such as changing how you think about the situation, changing how you feel about the situation, and problem-solving for solutions depending on the circumstances. You might:

- Call the interviewer to explain the situation and reschedule or switch to a virtual interview.
- Reframe your perspective by recognizing the situation is beyond your control and not your fault.
- Acknowledge that other opportunities will come along even if this one is lost.

To manage emotions, you can validate your frustration and reduce its intensity by reminding yourself that you did your best. You might turn on the AC, play relaxing music, or engage in deep breathing exercises to calm down.

Alternatively, you could resist reality, remain willful, and let the situation fuel your misery. Many of us have made this choice before, and perhaps some are doing so now.

Shared Struggles and Transformation

Radical acceptance reminds us that our pain, while deeply personal, is not unique. Countless others have faced similar struggles in health, relationships, careers, recreation, creativity, and purpose. There is comfort and validation in recognizing this shared human experience. You're not alone, and others have overcome similar challenges. This collective experience offers a path forward, a road map etched by those who have turned their pain into a path toward a new perspective, progress, and growth.

Take solace in imagining the countless individuals who have faced similar circumstances, initiated their journey toward healing, and emerged transformed. They've moved from chaos to harmony, reframing their struggles as pivotal moments of growth. Many have shifted their narratives from grief to gratitude, from feeling tattered and hopeless to becoming triumphant, filled with stories of resilience and renewal.

The Call to Transformation

Like those before you, you, too, can be part of this transformation. Radical acceptance calls us to step beyond ourselves, to discover untapped reservoirs of strength within the human spirit. Whether bowed but unbroken or broken yet reconstituted, you have the potential to join the ranks of those who have turned pain into purpose and meaning worth sharing. You can transform pain and suffering into a story of triumph, an alchemical process that reveals the resilient and boundless nature of the human soul.

Compassion

As we experience the process of transmutation and change through self-education and self-discovery, an unnerving grief may sink its talons into our psyche, its grip implacable; its grasp, irreconcilable. Such grief is the result of using an enlightened viewpoint to judge past behaviors and choices that were made in the dark. Subsequently, the ritual of psychological self-flagellation occurs as we begin engaging in a poisonous routine of self-blame, shame, guilt, and regret. We may internalize a myopic and punitive narrative that distorts a complete picture of the totality of our experiences. What we seek, what we need, is clemency. Who better to receive and express compassion than ourselves?

No matter how many books you read or adages you subscribe to, no matter how much compassion and validation you receive from others, nothing approaches the literal felt experience of being acquainted with your own slice of the human experience. Others may empathize, sympathize, and relate somewhat to the things you will inevitably go through, but no one, not even a perfectly crafted genetic clone of yourself, can truly know what it feels like to be you. This singularity of experience, while beautiful, can also feel isolating. Here lies the imperative for self-compassion, implemented with nonnegotiable and unyielding resolve.

As life inevitably tests the limits of our beliefs, behaviors, relationships, and emotions, we must remember: it is not a question of whether these trials will come, but when. Many of us have already endured profound pain, loss, and disappointment, wounds that defy expression even to ourselves, let alone to others. Inscribed onto the very fabric of human experience is the history of striving, survival, loss, disappointment, and yearning; of scratching and clawing for space, resources, peace, belonging, agency, safety, sanity, and solitude. And while we wait our turn on the conveyor belt moving us toward the unavoidable hamster wheel of pain, futility, and disappointment, we must take heart and have self-compassion.

Have self-compassion that this one pain cannot be avoided. Self-compassion for what it will do to you. Self-compassion that you will be changed by the experience. Self-compassion for your inner child and your current self and your inner elder. Self-compassion that you could barely protect yourself, let alone another. Self-compassion that you were scared, ashamed, craven. Self-compassion that you didn't know any better. Self-compassion that maybe you *thought* you knew better, but how could you have? If you had known this pain and suffering would be the outcome, you would certainly have made a different choice, taken a different path. Self-compassion that you were powerless in one situation or another. Self-compassion because this will not be the last time you will feel the pain and suffering inherent in being born in this world, in your body, in your family, your country, in this place, this time, this zeitgeist. This epoch. This moment. Self-compassion that no one gave you a blueprint, a map, a compass, the skills, the tools, the instruments you needed, and even if by some fortune someone did, they were rudimentary at best. Self-compassion that you did not know what questions to ask or what answers to give. And still, you are here. Reflecting. Learning. Transforming.

Self-compassion is not an indulgence; it is a necessity. It acknowledges the past without dwelling in it, offering grace, not because it erases pain, but because it serves as a salve to lessen the sting. Self-compassion is an act of quiet rebellion against the noises that demand perfection. It is a declaration, an exercise in dialectics: that you are enough, even as you strive to become more.

Expectations

We often spend much of our time hoping that things will unfold exactly as we expect. For some, that means anticipating the best; for others, fearing the worst. Yet, we often discount the infinite factors beyond our control that shape our daily experiences. Through a solipsistic lens, we convince ourselves that our singular agency is the primary force that moves the needle of our lives. This perspective, however, can lead to unnecessary suffering.

You expect a relationship to work, but despite your best efforts, it gradually fades as you and your partner reveal more of your true selves. You blame yourself or the other person, unwilling to acknowledge that circumstances evolve. You expect to fail a critical test and are paralyzed by anxiety, only to find yourself celebrating moments later when you pass. You have the qualifications for a job you were assured was all but yours, yet you're crushed when someone else is chosen. Or perhaps you pursue a career path you once believed would be financially fulfilling, only to feel the weight of doubt once you experience its emptiness. Or you train relentlessly in your sport or craft, only to taste the bitterness of defeat due to a single miscalculation. Could you have done more? Could you have done less?

Managing expectations is not about diminishing ambition or effort or being pessimistic, but about recognizing the unknowns in life and developing cognitive flexibility to counteract this truth. We are obligated to do our best with the information and skills we possess, but we need not engage in self-flagellation when reality unfolds in ways we did not anticipate, as it has, time and time again, yet we are still here. This is where the GRACE principles become essential: gratitude for what is, radical acceptance of what cannot be changed, and compassion, especially for ourselves when we feel the sting of unrealized expectations.

By practicing these principles, we cultivate the ability to manage expectations, remain present, reduce suffering, and experience eudaimonia more frequently.

Celebrating Success and Looking to the Future

A critical part of success is taking the time to celebrate your wins. Milestones and goals achieved offer a valuable opportunity to reflect on what you've accomplished. You deserve to pause, acknowledge yourself, and honor the collaborators and co-creators who helped you reach these benchmarks. Celebrating reinforces and rewards your hard work, the effective systems you created, and the consistency of your effort. No matter how you choose to celebrate, savor the moment in the eternal present and allow yourself to fully enjoy it.

Achieving your goals creates a ripple effect, inspiring those around you. Whether you serve as a role model, a mentor, or a source of quiet inspiration, your dedication and results do not go unnoticed. When you approach the world with a sense of transcendent purpose and raw authenticity, it becomes infectious. You may not always realize it, but both those close to you and strangers are observing, learning from, and emulating your actions and efforts.

To sustain your growth, it's essential to stay true to your values and principles. Building an aligned operating system, an ecosystem rooted in the integrity of your vision, is key. Like any new habit, setting and achieving your first few goals will require adjustment and adaptation. It will be challenging, and there will be moments when you feel like giving up. In those times, keep your eyes on the prize, the work will pay off, even when the process feels discouraging or overwhelming.

Pause and Reflect

Some reflection questions to help you on your HEART journey:

- Reflect on past changes or transitions in your life. How has your perception of them evolved over time, and what did you learn about yourself?
- Consider a specific setback or unexpected change. How did you manage it, and what lessons did you gain from the experience?
- Identify times in your life when you experienced flow. How did it enhance your well-being?
- What can you do routinely to create more opportunities for flow?
- Think about a goal you achieved. How did adaptability play a role, and what challenges did you overcome?
- Looking to the future, what new goals or transformations do you envision? How will you apply HEART, TRACE, and flow to them?
- What can you change to routinely have access to peace in your life?

Your Journey Forward

We've reached the end of our time together in this book. Take a moment to recognize the distance you've traveled. Reframing your life through the HEART approach and the guiding principles of TRACE processes is no small feat. It's a path paved with honesty, patience, and commitment. And here you are, standing on the foundation you've built, ready to move forward into a life that's truly meaningful.

My hope is that these pages have left you with renewed energy, clarity, and direction along with the confidence to make meaningful changes. These changes will serve you well in the interim as you work toward creating a life truly worth living.

Everything you've explored here is intended to help you begin your journey toward making real, lasting, positive changes in your life, and, by extension, in the lives of those around you. You've discovered the power of creating a framework through HEART priorities and TRACE processes, explored the characteristics of an autotelic personality, and learned how gratitude, self-acceptance, and compassion can act as forces of transformation.

But this isn't the end. It's only the beginning. You've now got a powerful framework, tools, insights, and values, that will guide you as you live in alignment with your deepest purpose. What living a purposeful life means is unique to each of us, but it always comes down to clarity, commitment, and the choice to act with intention every single day.

Embracing HEART as a Lifelong Ally

The HEART system isn't a fixed goal; it's a living, breathing ally that grows with you. It will evolve as your values shift and your aspirations change. In moments of challenge or transition, you now have the tools to pause, reassess, and recalibrate. HEART and TRACE can shift alongside you, supporting your growth as you navigate your journey with clarity and confidence.

Each element of HEART serves as a reminder of what's possible: health, enterprise, authentic relationships, recreation and recovery, and transcendent purpose and meaning, all working together. When these areas interconnect and reinforce one another, a rhythm emerges, a natural flow that keeps you grounded, aligned, and moving forward. As you continue on your path, returning to these areas regularly will become a practice of reflection, renewal, and course correction, especially when life inevitably shifts.

Start Your Next Chapter Today

Don't wait for the perfect moment to begin. Set a goal today, something simple yet meaningful. It could be a small habit or a goal for tomorrow. Use the TRACE processes to stay focused, even on the smaller steps. You'll discover that the act of regularly setting, revisiting, and expanding your goals is energizing in itself.

Adopting an autotelic mindset, the mindset that thrives on the process, will enrich your journey. Start each day with clarity, tuning into your values, and nurturing a centered approach. Embrace gratitude for the opportunities that arise and the people who walk alongside you. Reaffirm your commitment, stay open to feedback, and savor the freedom of choice as you build your path forward.

Although this marks the conclusion of your first read-through, I hope this book will serve as a lifelong guide and reference. Return to it whenever you need grounding, structure, confidence, or a refresher on the concepts we've covered. All the reflection exercises presented throughout the book have been compiled into a companion workbook called *Unselfing*. I hope you will try the workbook and find it useful as a tool to revisit your goals, practice self-reflection, and realign with your vision.

Share and Celebrate Your Journey

As you deepen your practice of this system, consider how your journey can ripple outward. Share your goals, seek mentorship, or even become a mentor yourself. Doing so allows you to connect with others, to uplift, and to be a source of encouragement, resilience, and inspiration. This is the beauty of living intentionally; it doesn't just transform you, it impacts everyone you encounter.

The way you live and approach life will leave an impression, showing others that purpose, personal growth, and fulfillment are within reach. Lean into those connections, because together, we rise.

Moving into a Purposeful Future

As you look ahead, know that this journey is ongoing. Life will continue to change, new challenges will arise, and new opportunities will present themselves. Each one is an invitation to apply what you've learned. With HEART and TRACE as your foundation, you are equipped to turn setbacks into lessons, to refine and adapt your goals, and to approach each new phase with intention and resolve.

This is your time. The future is yours to shape. With clarity, commitment, openness to challenge, and the power of choice, you're ready to create a future that aligns with your passions, your purpose, and the people who matter most to you.

Thank you for allowing me to be part of your journey. Now, go forward, live with purpose, and remember to celebrate each step along the way. I wish you all the best on your journey toward a eudaimonic life, a life of flourishing, meaning, and purpose.

Warmest wishes,

Dr. Ola Adenirange

*"You have not known what you are -- you have slumber'd
upon yourself all your life;
Your eye-lids have been the same as closed most of the time;
What you have done returns already in mockeries;
Your thrift, knowledge, prayers, if they do not return in
mockeries, what is their return?
The mockeries are not you;
Underneath them, and within them I see you lurk..."*

—EXCERPT FROM WALT WHITMAN'S POEM "TO YOU,"
FROM LEAVES OF GRASS.[30]

30   Whitman, Walt. "To You." In *Leaves of Grass*, 1856 ed. Brooklyn

Bibliography

American Psychological Association. APA Dictionary of Psychology (website), 2025. https://dictionary.apa.org/.

Duckworth, Angela. *Grit: The Power of Passion and Perseverance.* Scribner, 2016.

Jobs, Steve. "Steve Jobs' 2005 Stanford Commencement Address." Stanford University, June 12, 2005, posted March 7, 2008. YouTube, https://www.youtube.com/watch?v=UF8uR6Z6KLc/.

Jost, John T. (1995). Negative illusions: conceptual clarification and psychological evidence concerning false consciousness. *Political Psychology, 16*(2), 397–424. https://doi.org/10.2307/3791837

Kaushal, N., & Rhodes, R. E. (2015). Exercise habit formation in new gym members: A longitudinal study. *Journal of Behavioral Medicine, 38*(4), 652–663. https://doi.org/10.1007/s10865-015-9640-7

Kolk, Bessel van der. *The Body Keeps the Score: Brain, Mind, and Body in the Healing of Trauma.* Viking, 2014.

Lally, P., van Jaarsveld, C. H. M., Potts, H. W. W., & Wardle, J. (2010). How are habits formed: Modelling habit formation in the real world. *European Journal of Social Psychology, 40*(6), 998–1009. https://doi.org/10.1002/ejsp.674

Nhất Hạnh, Thích, *The Art of Living*. HarperCollins EPub Edition, June 2017. https://www.google.com/books/edition/The_Art_of_Living/97cIDAAAQBAJ/.

Pinker, Steven. "The Second Law of Thermodynamics." Edge.org, 2017. https://www.edge.org/response-detail/27023/.

Seneca, Lucius Annaeus (Seneca the Younger). *Stoic Philosophy of Seneca: Essays and Letters*. Edited by Moses Hadas. W.W. Norton, 1968.

Spencer, Maya. "What is spirituality?" Royal College of Psychiatrists, 2012. https://www.rcpsych.ac.uk/members/special-interest-groups/spirituality/publications-archive, section S, Dr Maya Spencer.

de Spinoza, Benedict. *Ethics, Part IV*. Translated by R.H.M. Elwes. Project Gutenberg, 2013. https://www.gutenberg.org/cache/epub/971/pg971-images.html.

Victor, Chitra G. Paul, and Judith V. Treschuk. "Critical Literature Review on the Definition Clarity of the Concept of Faith, Religion, and Spirituality." *Journal of Holistic Nursing*, 2019; vol. 38, iss. 1, pp. 107–113. doi:10.1177/0898010119895368.

About the Author

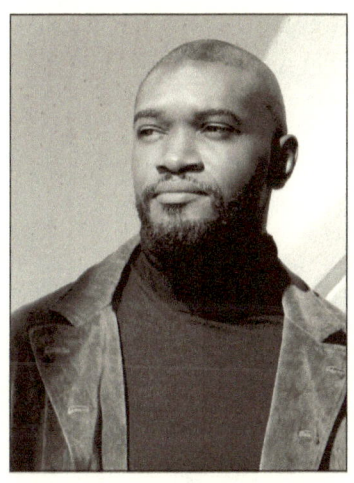

D r. Ola Adeniranye is a dually licensed psychologist, former U.S. Marine, and founder of Encomium Psychology, a clinical practice dedicated to helping individuals become self-possessed as they take on life's challenges with clarity, vigor, and vision. Grounded in evidence-based practice, philosophy, and lived experience, his work empowers others to create meaningful change and build a life of fulfillment and balance.

In his book *Unself: Transform Your Life By Letting Go of Who You're Not*, Dr. Adeniranye blends psychological insight with timeless wisdom as he explores the intersections of mental health, self-identity, and meaning in a rapidly evolving world. His positive, empowering system encourages readers to embrace growth, embody their values, and craft a life of intention and authenticity.

Beyond his professional work, Dr. Adeniranye finds excitement in the arts, literature, film, and music. He has a deep love for motorcycles and the freedom of the open road. He also cherishes time with his family and the experiences that come with travel, finding inspiration in new places, cultures, and perspectives. Whether immersed in a book, engaged in creative projects, or seeking adventure, he remains committed to both personal and collective transformation.

Connect with Dr. Ola here: https://www.encomiumpsychology.com/

Reviews

"Dr. Adeniranye has created a roadmap to happiness, helping readers shift from passive passengers to diligent drivers. He found clarity and awareness when he looked deeper and inward, sensing a calling to share with others how to live an authentic life. This book will invite you to seek more meaning in your life and give you answers to questions you never knew you had. If you are craving a more balanced life in a world full of noise, Dr. Adeniranye will give you the steps and tools to guide you through false consciousness, untethering the existential ghosts, and simplifying the complex search for happiness. If you want to break free from the unconscious chains and start living intentionally and with gratitude, this book will help you rewrite your narrative. This is a must-read for anyone who wants to taste the sweet nectar of happiness, being able to return to each passage at any point in their life and find fulfillment."
—**Dr. Amanda Moreno,** Psy.D.
Clinical Forensic Psychologist

"No pun intended, Dr. Ola cuts to the HEART of why many of us are unhappy, unfulfilled, and underwhelmed in life. Too often, people navigate through life on autopilot without a basic awareness of themselves and the things that matter most, such as health, relationships, values, purpose, and so on. This book challenges readers to take a deeper look at themselves, their ambitions, motivations, expectations, and the narratives for which they create and live by. Dr. Ola gives his readers the essential tools to help them explore their authentic selves and take meaningful action to aid their self-development by way of user-friendly acronyms and tools (HEART, TRACE, & GRACE). He also implores his audience to consider what may be getting in the way of true happiness without condemning or judging their choices. As a psychologist, I believe the information and tools offered in this

book will help my clients achieve true contentment and be more compassionate of themselves in the process. His user-friendly and no-nonsense approach makes this self-help book one worth delving into. Do yourself a favor and start your journey toward an authentic self."
—Dr. Antoine Saldubehere, Psy.D.
Psychologist In Private Practice, Specializing in Individual and Family Therapy

"Dr. Ola's UNSELF is a masterclass in personal transformation—clear, insightful, and deeply resonant. While the writing is incredibly accessible (you could technically read it in a couple of hours), to do so would be to miss the true magic of this book. This is not meant to be skimmed; it's meant to be lived with. It's a thoughtful, well-structured guide for those truly committed to inner work and lasting transformation; it's for those who are ready to slow down, dig deep, and engage with themselves on a much more meaningful level.

UNSELF is best experienced over time. Read a chapter a week. Pause. Reflect. Journal. Talk it through with friends or family. The book is intentionally designed to help you uncover the layers of who you're not, so you can reconnect with who you truly are. And if you give it that time and space, it will shift you. Not in some surface-level, feel-good way—but in the kind of way that makes you more honest, more clear, and more aligned.

There are no stories or fluff here—just clear, focused guidance and thoughtful prompts that help you take inventory of your patterns, assumptions, and internal blocks. Dr. Ola writes with a steady, grounded voice, gently nudging you toward greater self-awareness and freedom.

At its core, UNSELF is a guide to a more sustainable kind of happiness, "eudaimonic happiness" as the author notes—the kind that comes not from chasing external rewards, but from living in alignment with your values, your truth, and your purpose. It's about inner peace, clarity, and real growth.

In a world that often rewards performance over presence, UNSELF is a necessary and powerful invitation to come home to yourself."
—Talia Haller
Future of Health Thought Leader & Speaker

"I completely resonate with Dr. Ola's "HEART" concept. I'm constantly trying to illustrate the importance of this in a sociopolitical environment that overly emphasizes "safe spaces," "boundaries," and "protecting one's peace." These concepts, though well-intentioned, have created an illusion of health and can limit resilience, personal growth, and happiness. Dr. Ola's HEART concept I believe will help individuals break free from this illusion and subsequent fragility, to live more autonomous, competent, and connected lives for achieving and maintaining eudaimonia."
—Dr. Aileen Herlinda Sandoval, Psy.D.
Psychologist and Expert Witness on Brain Function and Autism Spectrum Disorder

"The Unself: Transforming Your Life by Letting Go of Who You're Not! written by Dr. Olabanji Adeniranye discusses different frameworks that will be helpful for individuals who may have difficulty understanding themselves, and how to transform their identity to their true selves.
Within the frameworks of HEART and TRACE, Dr. Ola explains the specificity of each aspect that an individual needs in order to work towards and maintain their true, authentic self. Utilizing HEART (Health, Enterprise, Authentic relationship, Recreation/recovery, and Transcendence Purpose) helps individuals understand why they think and act the way they do, and how to become better versions of themselves, using the strategies that TRACE provides (Time, Resistance, Awareness, Control, and Evolve). The concepts introduced in this book are simplified to help readers identify which areas they feel the need to improve, and which strategies to utilize as a process to accomplish their goals for personal growth.
As individuals, we tend to self-sabotage and have distorted perspectives of ourselves which lead us into a negative cycle of unhappiness and failure. In this book, Dr. Ola wants us to understand that even though it may seem normal to fail at certain things in life, that doesn't have to be the way we live our lives. There are many different perspectives and techniques we can use to not only transform and grow, but to continue to learn about ourselves and the potential of our future.

This book is well thought out and will help individuals identify areas that need improvement, and ways to accomplish their personal growth using these frameworks and perspectives."
—**Dr. Tania Hormozi,** PsyD, LMFT
Self-published Author, Cooked vs. Uncooked Spaghetti

www.ingramcontent.com/pod-product-compliance
Lightning Source LLC
Chambersburg PA
CBHW031316120626
46554CB00001BA/435